Atlas of the Human Body

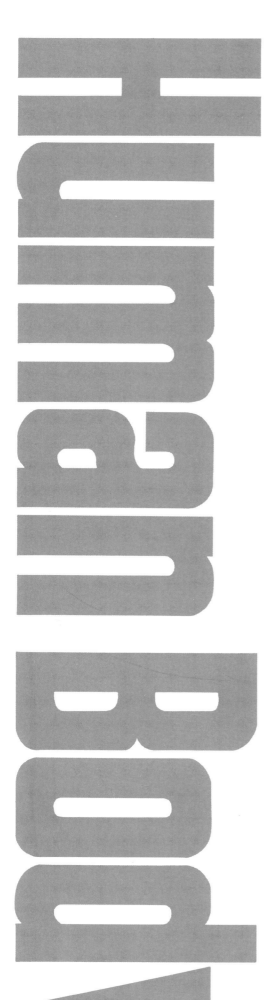

Atlas of the Human Body

HarperPerennial

A Division of HarperCollins*Publishers*

Some of the graphics and illustrations appearing in this book have been reproduced from *Encyclopedia of Medical Sciences, Cells and Tissues of the Human Body* and *The Human Body: A Practical Guide for Nurses*, all published by Kodansha.

Other original illustrations for this book were created by: Atsuto Onozawa, Katsusuke Saeki, Kazuyuki Chida, Satoaki Nikaidoh and Den Yamuchi.

Photographs in this book have been provided by the following people:
p. 13   3. Major maladies of the brain (2. Cerebral thrombosis) by Shunsaku Hirai
p. 13   3. Major maladies of the brain (3. Epidural hematoma) by Shogo Misawa
p. 15   3. The brain (2. Lateral surface, 3. Lower surface) by Akira Kanemitsu
p. 37   2. Alveoli and gas exchange (3. Sample mold of alveolar capillaries) by Takao Takizawa
p. 56   5. Inside of the stomach by Yukio Nagamachi
p. 56   6. Surface of the gastric mucous membrane viewed through a scanning electron microscope by Torao Yamamoto
p. 64   4. The liver is a mass of blood vessels—tissue molding model of blood vessels by Masahiko Machida
p. 74   2. Ureteral opening viewed through a cystoscope by Toyohei Machida
p. 117   3. Surface of skin viewed by a scanning electron microscope by Hiroyuki Suzuki
p. 119   6. Scalp and head viewed by a scanning electron microscope by Hiroyuki Suzuki

Book design/graphics layout by Noriko Shiga/Kohji Sugiura
English version design by Kim Llewellyn

This book was first published in Japan by Kodansha in 1989 under the title *Karada no Chizucho*.

HarperCollins books may be purchased for educational, business, or sales promotional use. For information, please write to: Special Markets Department, HarperCollins Publishers, Inc., 10 East 53rd Street, New York, N.Y. 10022.

FIRST EDITION

Library of Congress Cataloging-in-Publication Data

Karada no chizuchō. English.
    Atlas of the human body. — 1st ed.
      p. cm.
    First published: Japan : Kodansha, 1989.
    ISBN 0-06-273297-8 (pbk.)
    1. Human anatomy—Atlases. I. Title.
QM25.K3713 1994
611—dc20   94-4162

97 98   RRD   10 9 8 7 6 5

Preface

Questions: "How big is a kidney?" "Which one is located closer to the front of the neck, esophagus or trachea?" "What are the differences between subdural hemorrhage and subarchinoid hemorrhage?"

These questions are about our own bodies. However, many people seem to be unable to answer these questions correctly.

Whenever doctors attempt to explain to patients and their families about certain symptoms and necessary treatment or operation procedures for the symptoms, they, including myself, usually have to start the session by explaining how a human body is structured and how its organs function. In many cases, I felt it would be easier for patients and their families to understand these subjects if there were photographs or accurate graphics of internal organs. However, I believe there are few photographs available to serve this purpose. Many doctors frequently use simply drawn sketches of infected parts to explain the situation to their patients, but it is indeed difficult for patients to acquire a three-dimensional image of the body through a two-dimensional line drawing.

Some people have compared the human body to a microcosm because of the body's intricate structure, mysterious functions, strict regularity and harmonized activities, which some may call the divine creation. The human body is indeed a subject that would suit the image of mysterious microcosm, but it is not something that exists somewhere far away in space.

The first step in understanding this microcosm is to learn which parts of the body each organ is located in, and what kinds of functions each have. That is, to understand the mapping, or geography, of the body. While almost all persons have maps in their homes of the area in which they live, few possess maps or atlases of the human body.

This book is structured to give readers a general and comprehensive view of the human body. Readers can take it along on doctor appointments and have their personal physicians explain the symptoms, pointing at certain graphics in this book. After that, readers might carefully re-read the explanation in the parts that their doctor pointed out. I believe this kind of usage will help readers gain an accurate and necessary understanding of the body's geography.

Today, massive amounts of intelligence are employed to solve mysteries of the human body. New opinions and theories are added daily to the cutting-edge medical fields, creating active discussions and arguments that sometimes topple existing theories. During the editorial process, I intended to select subjects and theories that have been generally agreed upon but I still fear that there might be a point or two that may have been missed. For that reason, I welcome readers' opinions and criticism.

Finally, I would like to express my appreciation to Dr. Akio Yamauchi of Tokyo University, who extended generous assistance in the production of the graphics appearing in this book.

Takeo Takahashi

Contents

The Circulatory Organs

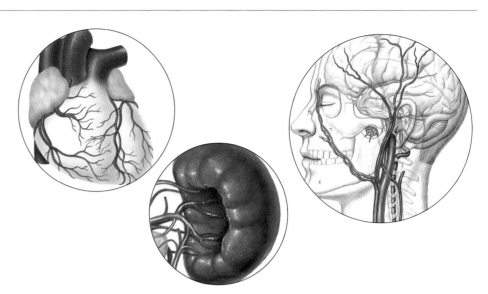
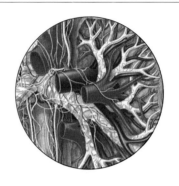
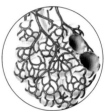

The Respiratory Organs

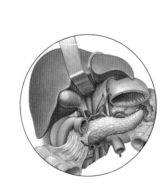

The Digestive Organs

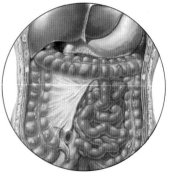

The Urinary and Reproductive Organs

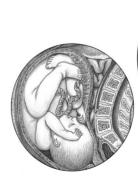
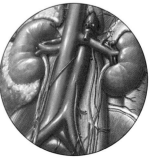

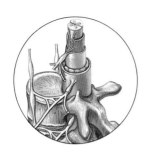
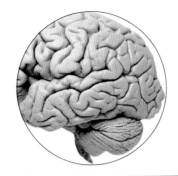

The Brain and Nerves

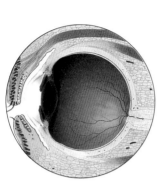
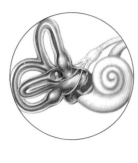

The Sensory Organs

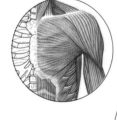
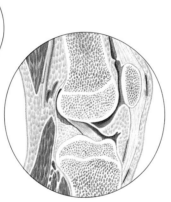

The Muscles and Bones

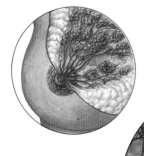
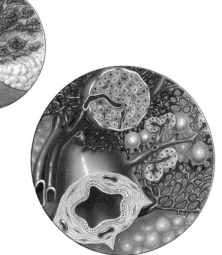

The Endocrine Organs

Using This Book—
Planes, Directions, and Parts of the Body

Right and left when used in explanations of the diagrams in this book refer to the right and left of the patient, not as it is viewed on the printed page.

MAIN BODY PLANES AND DIRECTIONS

Terms used in this book are defined below:

Median sagittal plane: a plane that divides an erect standing individual into left and right along a midline longitudinal plane. A plane which lies parallel to the median sagittal plane is referred to as a sagittal plane.

Transverse plane: a plane that divides an individual standing erect into upper and lower portions.

Frontal plane: a plane that divides an individual standing erect into dorsal and ventral portions.

Superior: refers to the upper area close to the head of an individual standing erect.

Inferior: refers to the lower area close to the lower limbs of an individual standing erect.

Ventral: refers to the chest and abdominal side. Anterior may also be used.

Dorsal: refers to the lumbar side. Posterior may also be used. When talking about the hand, it refers to the dorsum manus.

Deep: refers to the direction moving toward the midline, longitudinal plane.

Superficial: refers to the direction moving away from the midline, longitudinal plane.

Radial: refers to the direction moving toward the radius on the upper limbs (thumb side).

Ulnar: refers to the direction moving toward the ulna (fifth finger side).

Palmar: refers to the palm of the hand.

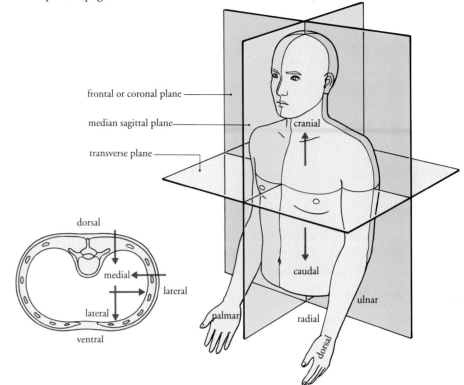

THE MAIN REGIONS OF THE BODY

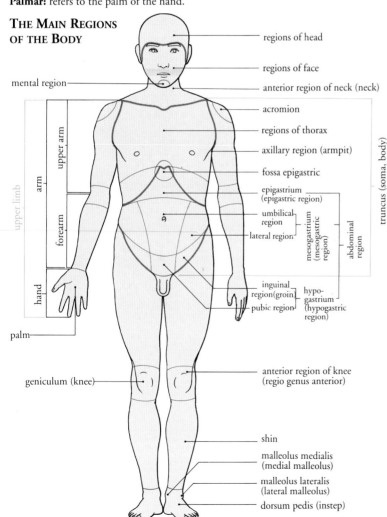

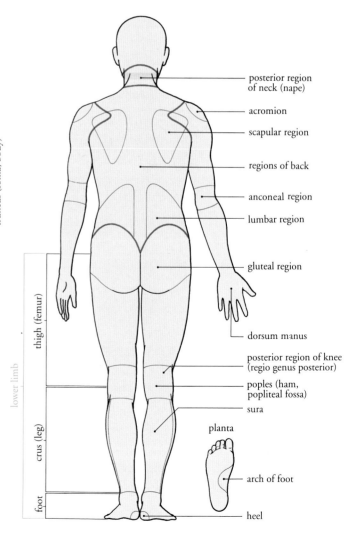

8

I The Head and Neck

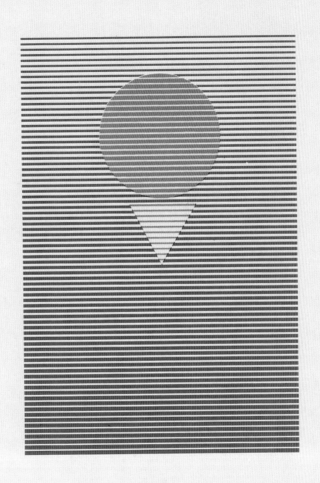

The Head and Neck

1. GENERAL VIEW OF THE HEAD AND NECK

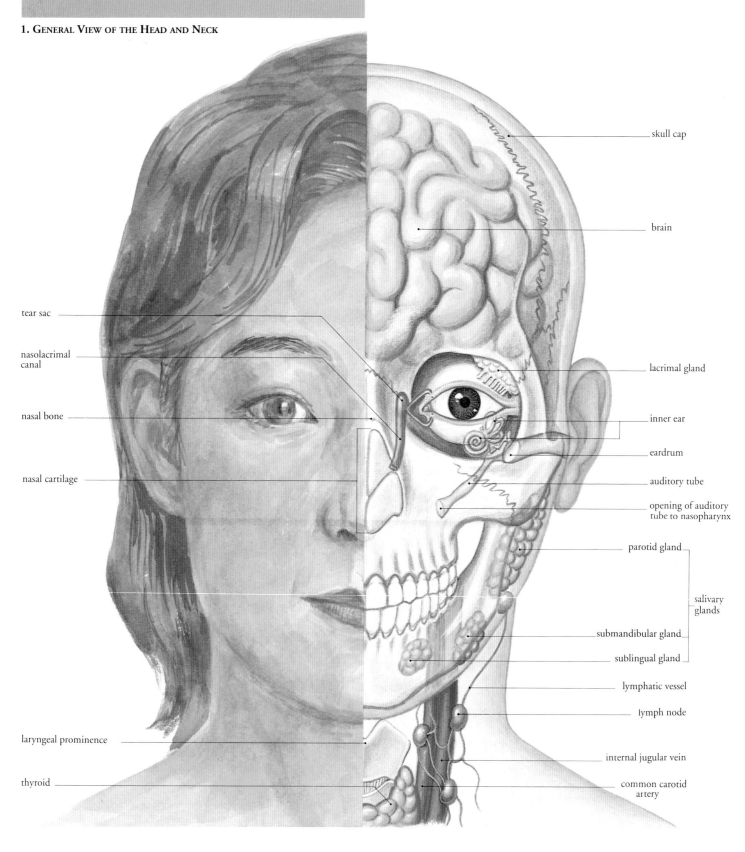

skull cap

brain

tear sac

nasolacrimal canal

nasal bone

nasal cartilage

lacrimal gland

inner ear

eardrum

auditory tube

opening of auditory tube to nasopharynx

parotid gland

salivary glands

submandibular gland

sublingual gland

lymphatic vessel

lymph node

laryngeal prominence

internal jugular vein

thyroid

common carotid artery

The head is the place where nerve activity occurs, the command center for the entire body. It is also the region where the major sensory organs are located. The most elaborate and individual capabilities found in the human body are stored here.

Inside the cranial skull are the cerebrum, which performs high level nerve activity; the cerebellum, which controls the subtle body actions responding to commands from the cerebrum; and the brain stem, which coordinates the activity necessary for such

life-sustaining functions as breathing and circulation of blood.

The front part of the skull, composed of facial bones, houses the sensory organs, including the eyes, ears, nose, and tongue, which perceive changes outside the body. The expressive muscles, which indicate joy and sadness, for example, are attached here, making the face the stage for displaying emotional states.

The neck, which connects the head to the body, supports the weight of the head through the cervical spine and muscles; the

1. Magnification of the Subarachnoid Space

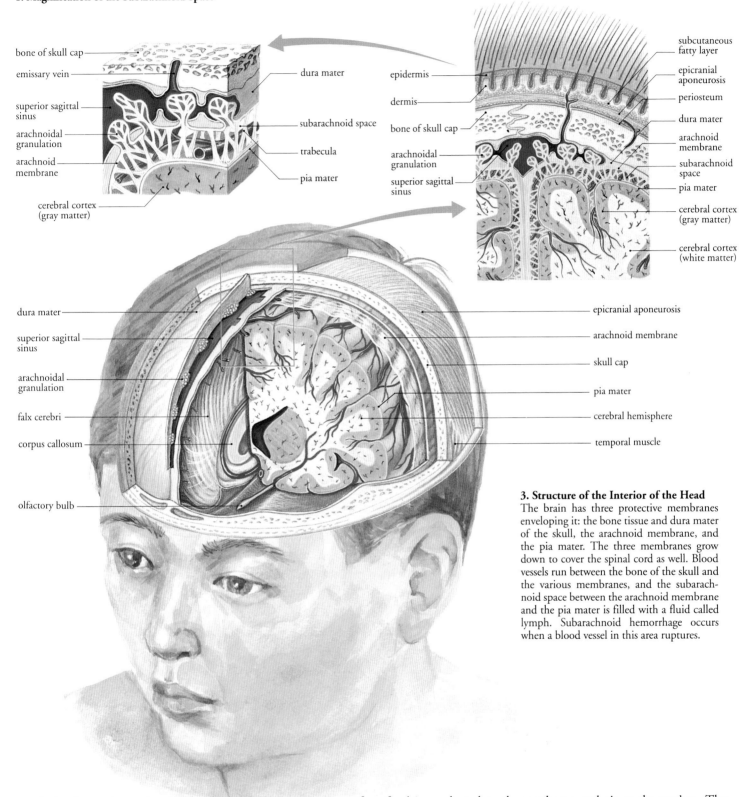

bone of skull cap

emissary vein

superior sagittal sinus

arachnoidal granulation

arachnoid membrane

cerebral cortex (gray matter)

dura mater

subarachnoid space

trabecula

pia mater

epidermis

dermis

bone of skull cap

arachnoidal granulation

superior sagittal sinus

subcutaneous fatty layer

epicranial aponeurosis

periosteum

dura mater

arachnoid membrane

subarachnoid space

pia mater

cerebral cortex (gray matter)

cerebral cortex (white matter)

dura mater

superior sagittal sinus

arachnoidal granulation

falx cerebri

corpus callosum

olfactory bulb

epicranial aponeurosis

arachnoid membrane

skull cap

pia mater

cerebral hemisphere

temporal muscle

3. Structure of the Interior of the Head

The brain has three protective membranes enveloping it: the bone tissue and dura mater of the skull, the arachnoid membrane, and the pia mater. The three membranes grow down to cover the spinal cord as well. Blood vessels run between the bone of the skull and the various membranes, and the subarachnoid space between the arachnoid membrane and the pia mater is filled with a fluid called lymph. Subarachnoid hemorrhage occurs when a blood vessel in this area ruptures.

cervical spine and muscles also make possible free movement of the head. Nerves, including the spinal cord, pass through the cervical region. Commands originating in the central nervous system (cerebrum, cerebellum, brain stem) and information from the body and limbs pass to the brain through this region. Thick arteries supplying oxygen and energy and large veins and lymph vessels carrying out waste also pass through this region.

The cervical region also houses the pharynx, through which food is conducted to the esophagus and air to the trachea. The epiglottis, which protects the trachea by allowing only gaseous bodies and steam to pass into the trachea, and the larynx, containing the vocal cords, are also in the cervical region, as is the body's largest endocrine gland, the thyroid, found in the anterior part of the cervical region.

The Skull and Blood Vessels of the Head

SKULL

The bony framework of the head protects the central nervous system of the brain, as well as the eyes, nose, ears, and other major sensory organs from traumatic injury.

The skull is divided into the cranial bones and facial bones. The cranial bones are the frontal bone, occipital bone, sphenoid bone, ethmoid bone, a pair of temporal bones (one each on the left and right side), and parietal bones. The seams joining these bones are wavy, resembling lines of a jigsaw puzzle. The patterns of these seams are finer in the female skull than in the male. In the fetus, the parts in the immediate area of the seams are still cartilage, hence flexible, enabling the skull to narrow temporarily and pass through the thick birth canal during delivery.

Parts of the thick frontal, maxillary, and sphenoid bones are hollow, making the skull lighter. The temporal bones are relatively thin and thus break more easily than other bones in the skull.

ARTERIES AND VEINS OF THE HEAD AND NECK

If you move your finger from the side of the base of the neck toward the front, you will feel the pulse of the common carotid artery. The two common carotid arteries, which are found on either side of the neck, divide into the external carotid artery and the internal carotid artery as they near the jawbone. The external carotid arteries mainly supply blood to the tissues outside the skull. The left and right internal carotid arteries join the vertebral artery to form a ring at the base of the brain, and from there divide into three pairs of arteries to supply blood to various tissues of the central nervous system in the skull, including the arachnoid membrane, cerebrum, and cerebellum.

Brain tissue has end arteries. In other parts of the body, arteries are usually connected to other nearby arteries, but in the case of the end artery, a single artery supplies the blood. As a result, if an end artery ruptures or becomes clogged, the region supplied by that artery is immediately deprived of blood and suffers irreparable damage.

On the facial side, although there are numerous blood vessels, there is very little tissue to act as a cushion between the skin and bone, so a blow to this area can easily rupture blood vessels to cause bleeding.

Major Disorders: Cerebral infarction, cerebral thrombosis, cerebral hemorrhage, subarachnoid hemorrhage, transient ischemic attack, etc.

1. SKULL

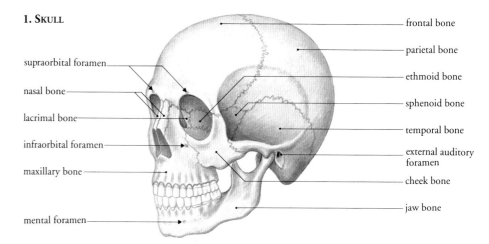

frontal bone
parietal bone
ethmoid bone
sphenoid bone
temporal bone
external auditory foramen
cheek bone
jaw bone

supraorbital foramen
nasal bone
lacrimal bone
infraorbital foramen
maxillary bone
mental foramen

1. Front Diagonal View of the Skull

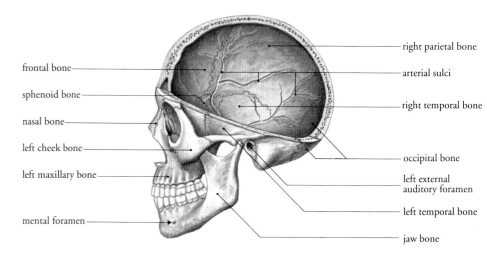

right parietal bone
arterial sulci
right temporal bone
occipital bone
left external auditory foramen
left temporal bone
jaw bone

frontal bone
sphenoid bone
nasal bone
left cheek bone
left maxillary bone
mental foramen

2. Interior of the Temporal Region
Important blood vessels form grooves passing the underside of the temporal bones. This is the reason injury to the temporal region of the head can easily rupture blood vessels and cause serious damage. To show the grooves, this illustration omits the blood vessels.

front

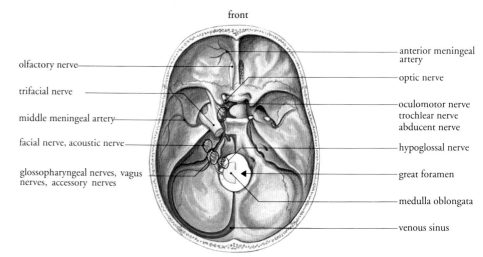

olfactory nerve
trifacial nerve
middle meningeal artery
facial nerve, acoustic nerve
glossopharyngeal nerves, vagus nerves, accessory nerves

anterior meningeal artery
optic nerve
oculomotor nerve
trochlear nerve
abducent nerve
hypoglossal nerve
great foramen
medulla oblongata
venous sinus

3. Interior of the Base of the Skull
Horizontal section viewed from the base of the forehead. The left half shows the nerves and blood vessels entering and exiting the skull. The right half shows only the routes (arterial foramina) they travel.

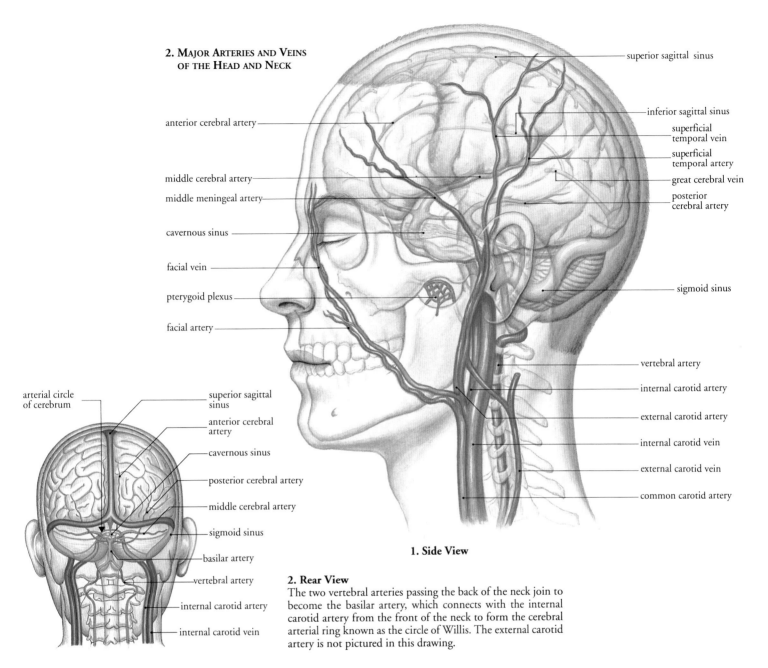

2. Major Arteries and Veins of the Head and Neck

superior sagittal sinus

inferior sagittal sinus

superficial temporal vein

superficial temporal artery

great cerebral vein

posterior cerebral artery

sigmoid sinus

vertebral artery

internal carotid artery

external carotid artery

internal carotid vein

external carotid vein

common carotid artery

anterior cerebral artery

middle cerebral artery

middle meningeal artery

cavernous sinus

facial vein

pterygoid plexus

facial artery

arterial circle of cerebrum

superior sagittal sinus

anterior cerebral artery

cavernous sinus

posterior cerebral artery

middle cerebral artery

sigmoid sinus

basilar artery

vertebral artery

internal carotid artery

internal carotid vein

1. Side View

2. Rear View
The two vertebral arteries passing the back of the neck join to become the basilar artery, which connects with the internal carotid artery from the front of the neck to form the cerebral arterial ring known as the circle of Willis. The external carotid artery is not pictured in this drawing.

3. Major Maladies of the Brain

1. Brain Aneurysm (arrow)

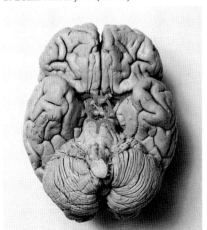

Often forms in the circle of Willis at the base of the brain. If it ruptures, sub-arachnoid hemorrhage occurs.

2. Cerebral Thrombosis

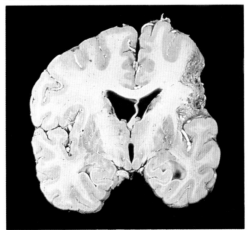

Illustration of a brain in which one part has suffered softening as a result of blockage of blood vessels from a cerebral thrombosis.

3. Epidural Hematoma

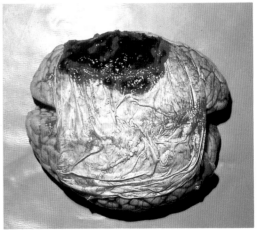

Hematoma formed between the skull and the dura mater owing to ruptured blood vessels resulting from an external injury to the head.

13

The Brain and Spinal Cord

- **Cerebrum:** length: approx 16–18 cm, width: approx 12–14 cm, weight: males, approx 1350 g; females, approx 1250 g.
- **Cerebellum:** average weight: males 135 g; females 122 g.
- **Spinal Cord:** length: approx 44 cm, diameter: approx 1–1.5 cm, weight: approx 25 g.

BRAIN

Enclosed in the skull the brain comprises the cerebrum and cerebellum, which envelop the brain stem.

Cerebrum. In the adult male the cerebrum weighs approx 1350 g; in the adult female, approx 1250 g. It is divided into left and right hemispheres by the longitudinal cerebral fissure. A cortex (gray matter) 2–5 mm thick covers the medullary substance (white matter). Three thin membranes, the dura mater, arachnoid membrane and pia mater, envelop the cortex. The cortex is gray with a pinkish cast caused by the collection of nerve cells, and is patterned with undulations. The white matter is the collection of nerve fibers from the nerve cells; inside the white matter is the mass of nerve cells known as the basal nuclei (basal ganglia).

The cerebral cortex is phylogenetically divided into the neocortex, archicortex, and paleocortex. In humans and primates the archicortex and paleocortex are covered by the well-developed neocortex and cannot be seen from the surface. The neocortex controls advanced mental activities. The archicortex and paleocortex, with the basal nuclei, form the functional unit called the limbic system, which is the center of reflex movement, emotions, and memory.

Brain Stem. The brain stem is the part of the brain, resembling a guppy in shape, that connects the cerebral hemispheres to the spinal cord. The diencephalon, mesencephalon, pons, and medulla oblongata are arranged in that order from top to bottom. At the end of a stem, extending from the diencephalon, hangs the hypophysis, or pituitary gland, which is small in size but controls the body's hormones.

Broadly divided into the thalamus and hypothalamus, the diencephalon is a collection of numerous nuclei (clusters of nerve cells). The red nucleus and nigra, which are related to movement, are located in the mesencephalon. In the central area of the mesencephalon and spinal cord is found the reticular formation made up of nerve cells and fibers connected in a net-like form; this is involved in coordinating muscle movement, consciousness, and vigilance. As a whole, the brain stem is the center of such vital life functions as respiration, heart function, and temperature adjustment.

Cerebellum. Located on the back of the pons and medulla oblongata, the cerebellum is almost completely hidden by the temporal lobes of the cerebral hemispheres. In the adult male it weighs approx 135 g; in the adult female, approx 122 g. The central portion is an oval hemisphere with a canal running across the surface. It is the center for maintaining the body's balance and acts as the receptor of signals from the sensory organs of the skin and muscles. It is also responsible for coordinating muscle movement.

Major Disorders: brain tumor, Japanese encephalopathy, etc.

1. STRUCTURE OF THE BRAIN

1. Cross Section of Brain

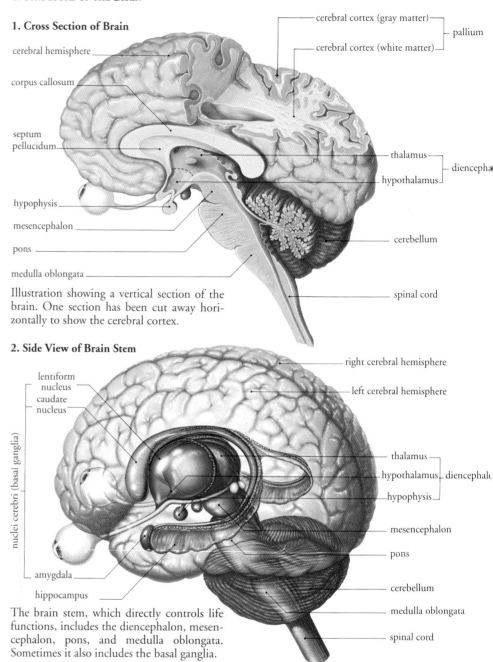

Illustration showing a vertical section of the brain. One section has been cut away horizontally to show the cerebral cortex.

Labels: cerebral hemisphere; corpus callosum; septum pellucidum; hypophysis; mesencephalon; pons; medulla oblongata; cerebral cortex (gray matter); cerebral cortex (white matter); pallium; thalamus; hypothalamus; diencephalon; cerebellum; spinal cord

2. Side View of Brain Stem

The brain stem, which directly controls life functions, includes the diencephalon, mesencephalon, pons, and medulla oblongata. Sometimes it also includes the basal ganglia.

Labels: nuclei cerebri (basal ganglia); lentiform nucleus; caudate nucleus; amygdala; hippocampus; right cerebral hemisphere; left cerebral hemisphere; thalamus; hypothalamus; diencephalon; hypophysis; mesencephalon; pons; cerebellum; medulla oblongata; spinal cord

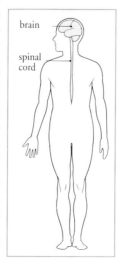

brain; spinal cord

2. FUNCTIONS OF THE CEREBRUM

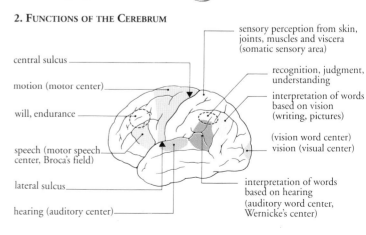

The functions of the cerebrum differ by area. This drawing of the exterior of the cerebrum illustrates where each function is located.

Labels: central sulcus; motion (motor center); will, endurance; speech (motor speech center, Broca's field); lateral sulcus; hearing (auditory center); sensory perception from skin, joints, muscles and viscera (somatic sensory area); recognition, judgment, understanding; interpretation of words based on vision (writing, pictures); (vision word center) vision (visual center); interpretation of words based on hearing (auditory word center, Wernicke's center)

3. THE BRAIN

1. Upper Surface

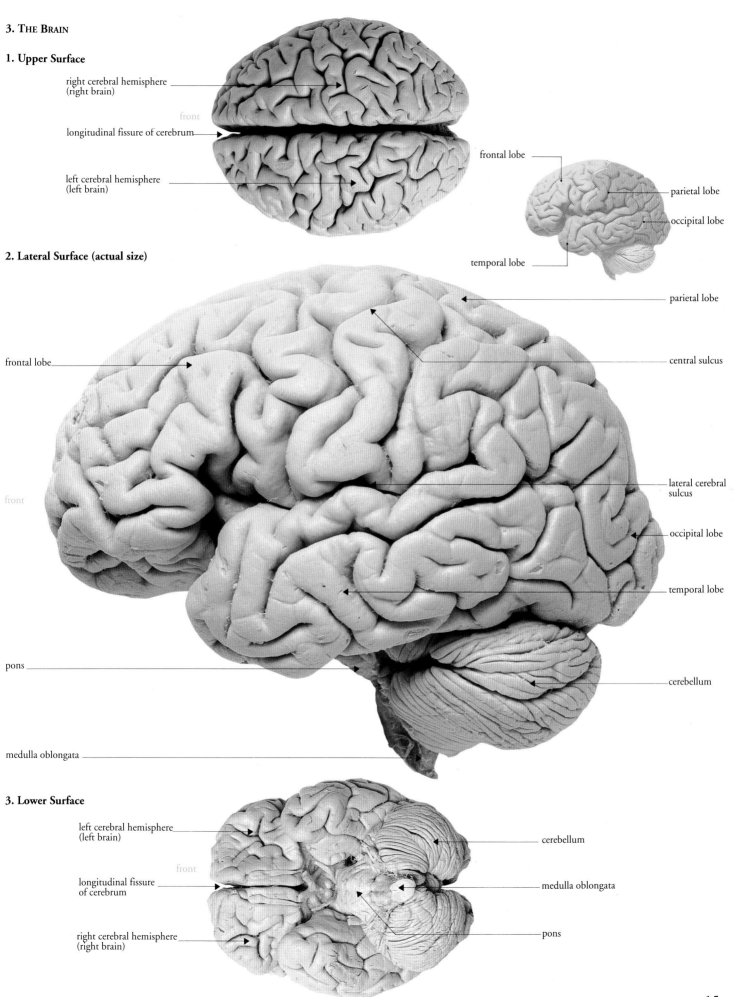

right cerebral hemisphere (right brain)

longitudinal fissure of cerebrum

left cerebral hemisphere (left brain)

frontal lobe

parietal lobe

occipital lobe

temporal lobe

2. Lateral Surface (actual size)

front

frontal lobe

parietal lobe

central sulcus

lateral cerebral sulcus

occipital lobe

temporal lobe

pons

cerebellum

medulla oblongata

3. Lower Surface

left cerebral hemisphere (left brain)

front

longitudinal fissure of cerebrum

right cerebral hemisphere (right brain)

cerebellum

medulla oblongata

pons

THE SPINAL CORD

The spinal cord is a long bundle of nerve fibers that acts as a center for reflex actions as well as the pathway to and from the brain for nervous impulses.

Location. The spinal cord extends approx two-thirds of the way down the back from the medulla oblongata in the head. In the adult human it is approx 44 cm long and weighs approx 25 g. It is enclosed within a ring of bone formed by the vertebral bodies (corpus vertebrae). Together the vertebrae make up a protective tunnel for the spinal cord called the vertebral canal. The spinal cord ends with the terminus of the narrow roots descending from the conus medullaris. The spinal nerves extending from the upper part of the conus medullaris resemble the tail of a horse. Hence, this part is called the cauda equina.

Structure. Like the brain, the spinal cord is covered by three membranes, the dura mater, the arachnoid membrane, and the pia mater. Collectively, these membranes are called the spinal meninges (singula meninx). When the spinal cord is cut crosswise, it can be seen that (in contrast to the cerebrum and cerebellum) the outer substance—the white matter—surrounding the inner substance—the gray matter—is in the shape of the letter "H." The white matter comprises mainly the axons (see p. 126), whereas the gray matter is mainly neurons (see p. 126, Nerve Cells and Their Short Dendric Processes and Axons). The anterior section of the "H" is called the anterior grayhorn (cornu anterius) and the posterior section is called the posterior grayhorn (cornu posterius). The neurons of the anterior grayhorn are primarily related to movement and connected to the motor nerves, and the neurons of the posterior grayhorn are mainly involved in sensation and joined to the somesthetic nerves (sensory nerves). The part of the "H" where the middle bar intersects the sides is called the cornu lateralis, and the neurons of this part are connected to the sympathetic nerves.

Function. The spinal cord acts as the pathway for nerve signals to and from the brain, including the brain stem, and the various parts of the body. Signals from outside the body are communicated via this pathway to the brain, which in turn sends out the proper commands to the arms, legs, or other parts of the body. In urgent or dangerous situations reflex actions take over, foregoing communication to the brain. In such cases, the spinal cord functions as the command center. The spinal cord also controls the internal organs and blood vessels, acting as the center for involuntary reflexes.

Major Disorders: spinal cord injury, amyotrophic lateral sclerosis, syringomyelia, spinal cord tumor, meningitis.

4. GENERAL VIEW OF THE SPINAL CORD

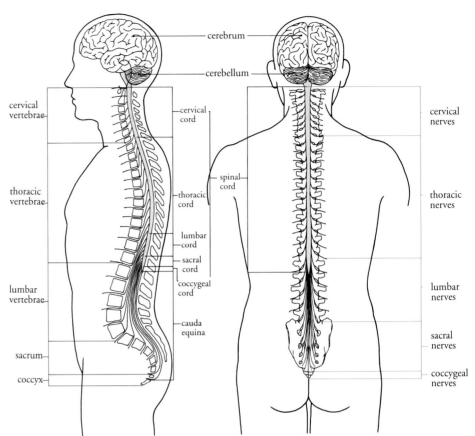

The Parts of the Spinal Cord and the Relationship Between the Backbone and the Spinal Nerves

5. FUNCTIONS OF THE SPINAL CORD

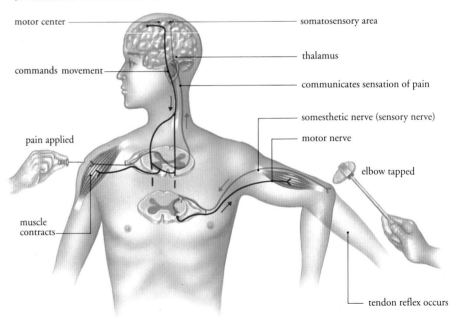

The spinal cord acts as the pathway for nerve signals connecting the various parts of the body and the brain. The left side of this illustration shows a message from outside the body being communicated to the brain and the brain's response (command to the muscle to contract). Both of these impulses are relayed via the spinal cord. It also serves as a command center for reflex actions. The right side of the illustration shows the spinal cord acting as the nerve center and commanding an involuntary reflex.

6. STRUCTURE OF THE SPINAL CORD

1. Three-Dimensional Model of the Spinal Cord

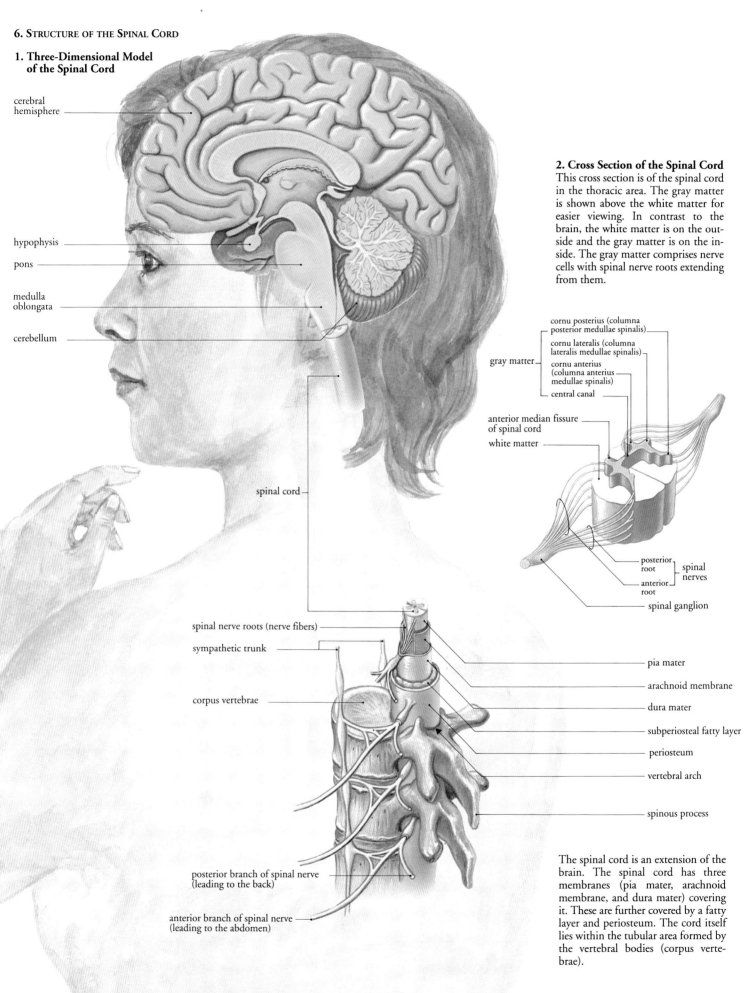

cerebral hemisphere

hypophysis

pons

medulla oblongata

cerebellum

spinal cord

2. Cross Section of the Spinal Cord

This cross section is of the spinal cord in the thoracic area. The gray matter is shown above the white matter for easier viewing. In contrast to the brain, the white matter is on the outside and the gray matter is on the inside. The gray matter comprises nerve cells with spinal nerve roots extending from them.

gray matter

cornu posterius (columna posterior medullae spinalis)

cornu lateralis (columna lateralis medullae spinalis)

cornu anterius (columna anterius medullae spinalis)

central canal

anterior median fissure of spinal cord

white matter

posterior root
anterior root
} spinal nerves

spinal ganglion

pia mater

arachnoid membrane

dura mater

subperiosteal fatty layer

periosteum

vertebral arch

spinous process

spinal nerve roots (nerve fibers)

sympathetic trunk

corpus vertebrae

posterior branch of spinal nerve (leading to the back)

anterior branch of spinal nerve (leading to the abdomen)

The spinal cord is an extension of the brain. The spinal cord has three membranes (pia mater, arachnoid membrane, and dura mater) covering it. These are further covered by a fatty layer and periosteum. The cord itself lies within the tubular area formed by the vertebral bodies (corpus vertebrae).

17

The Eye

- Average diameter approx 24 mm
- Distance front to back approx 23–25 mm

1. THE EYE AND ACCESSORY STRUCTURES

Tears produced in the lacrimal gland flow through the excretory ducts to the eye to wet the surface of the eyeball. Tears then pass into the lacrimal punctum and tear sac and through the lower nasal passage. This explains why weeping is accompanied by a runny nose.

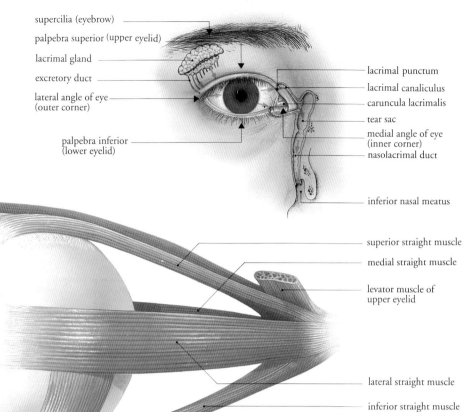

supercilia (eyebrow)
palpebra superior (upper eyelid)
lacrimal gland
excretory duct
lateral angle of eye (outer corner)
palpebra inferior (lower eyelid)
lacrimal punctum
lacrimal canaliculus
caruncula lacrimalis
tear sac
medial angle of eye (inner corner)
nasolacrimal duct
inferior nasal meatus

2. MUSCLES THAT MOVE THE EYEBALL (LEFT EYE)

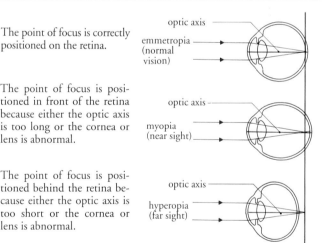

superior oblique muscle
inferior oblique muscle
superior straight muscle
medial straight muscle
levator muscle of upper eyelid
lateral straight muscle
inferior straight muscle

3. PATHWAYS TO THE VISUAL CENTERS OF THE CEREBRUM

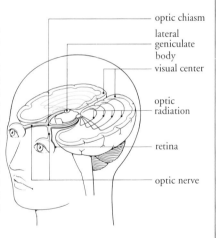

Visual information from the external environment is turned into electric signals in the retina and sent to the optic nerves. Some of the fibers of the optic nerve from each eye cross each other in the middle at the optic chiasm. The electric signals then pass along the optic tract to the lateral geniculate body and optic radiations to the visual center of the cerebral cortex, giving rise to the sense of sight.

optic chiasm
lateral geniculate body
visual center
optic radiation
retina
optic nerve

4. NORMAL AND ABNORMAL REFRACTION

The point of focus is correctly positioned on the retina.

The point of focus is positioned in front of the retina because either the optic axis is too long or the cornea or lens is abnormal.

The point of focus is positioned behind the retina because either the optic axis is too short or the cornea or lens is abnormal.

optic axis
emmetropia (normal vision)

optic axis
myopia (near sight)

optic axis
hyperopia (far sight)

The eye receives information from light. In humans, 80% of information is perceived by the eye.

Location and Size. The eyeball, cushioned in a layer of fat, is located inside a protective socket within the skull. The eyeball is formed by two spherical bodies of different sizes that are attached to each other. The anterior chamber and the cornea make up the smaller sphere. The larger sphere is called the posterior chamber (vitreous chamber) and is enveloped by the sclera. The average diameter of a normal eyeball of an adult human is 24 mm, and the distance from front to back is about 23-25 mm.

Structure and Function. The eye is like a camera. The cornea protects the lens and acts as a colorless filter to refract light. The lens of the eye is flexible, changing thickness in response to the contraction and relaxation of the ciliary muscles. The lens becomes thin to help focus on distant objects, and when the muscles relax, the lens becomes thick to help bring nearby objects into focus. The role of the lens is to make subtle adjustments in focusing light on the retina. The iris corresponds to the aperture in a camera, controlling the amount of light that enters the eye. The vitreous body is a gelatinous substance within the vitreous chamber that maintains the shape of the eye. Intraocular fluid called aque-

5. STRUCTURE OF THE EYE

1. Cross Section of the Eye Socket

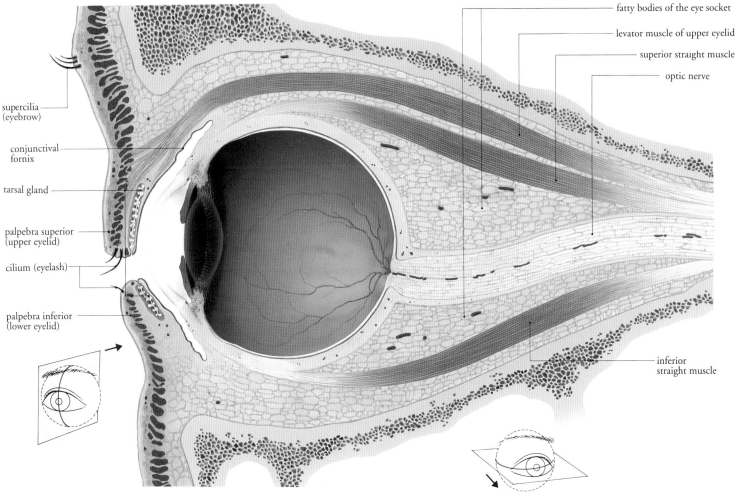

fatty bodies of the eye socket

levator muscle of upper eyelid

superior straight muscle

optic nerve

supercilia (eyebrow)

conjunctival fornix

tarsal gland

palpebra superior (upper eyelid)

cilium (eyelash)

palpebra inferior (lower eyelid)

inferior straight muscle

2. Circulatory Route of Aqueous Humor

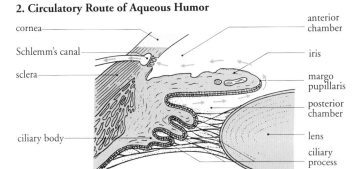

cornea

Schlemm's canal

sclera

ciliary body

anterior chamber

iris

margo pupillaris

posterior chamber

lens

ciliary process

Aqueous humor is secreted from the ciliary body. The fluid passes through the posterior and anterior chambers and enters Schlemm's canal. If the flow of aqueous humor is blocked, intraocular pressure increases, resulting in glaucoma. Arrows indicate the direction of flow of this fluid.

ous humor supplies nourishment to the eyes.

The retina corresponds to the film of a camera: The images are projected onto it and then changed into electric signals. The visual cells of the retina include rods and cones. Rods are sensitive to changes in light but not color, whereas cones perceive color. Each visual cell is connected to a nerve fiber, all of which combine to form the optic nerve. The optic nerve relays signals to the visual center of the cerebrum, giving rise to vision.

The Muscles That Move the Eyeball. Three pairs of muscles are attached to each eyeball. The eyes move in coordination when focusing on an object.

3. Horizontal Section of Eyeball (right eye)

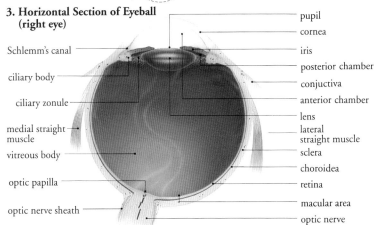

pupil

cornea

iris

posterior chamber

conjuctiva

anterior chamber

lens

lateral straight muscle

sclera

choroidea

retina

macular area

optic nerve

Schlemm's canal

ciliary body

ciliary zonule

medial straight muscle

vitreous body

optic papilla

optic nerve sheath

Lacrimal Glands and Tears. The lacrimal gland produces tears and resembles an almond in size and shape. It is located slightly above the eyeball on the inner side of the eye socket and close to the outer corner of the eye. Tears contain a substance that kills bacteria, they act as a lubricant between the eyelid and the cornea, and they flood foreign matter out of the eye. In addition, tears help express emotions, such as sadness and frustration.

Major Disorders: abnormal refraction (farsightedness, nearsightedness, astigmatism, presbyopia), color blindness, strabismus, inflammation (conjunctivitis, uveitis), abnormal intraocular pressure (glaucoma), cataract, retinodialysis, external injury.

The Ear

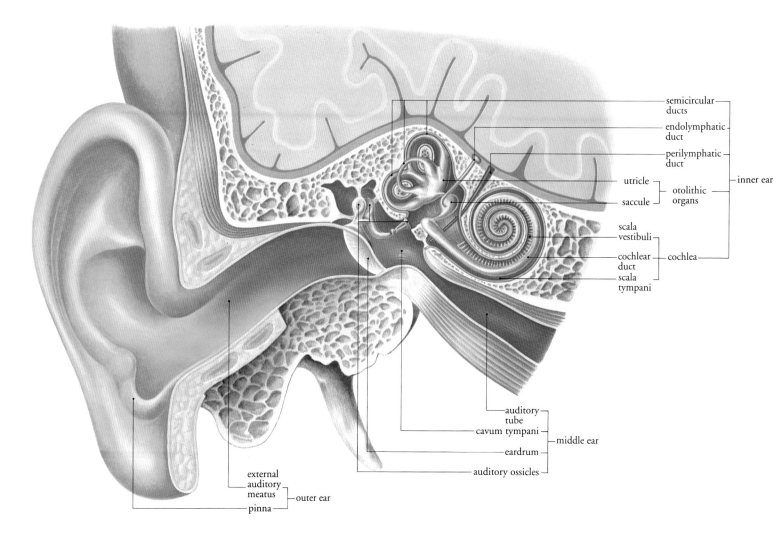

The ear governs hearing and balance. The ear includes the pinna (the outer cartilaginous structure), the auditory organs (hearing), and the vestibula organs (balance) made up of the semicircular ducts, utricle, and saccule. Only the pinna and part of the external auditory meatus can be seen from the outside.

The Auditory Organs of the Ear. Air passing through the external auditory meatus causes the eardrum between the outer ear and the middle ear to vibrate. The eardrum is a thin membrane shaped like a cone with the concave side facing the opening of the external auditory meatus. Just behind the eardrum are three bones called the auditory ossicles: the hammer (malleus) and anvil (incurst) bones serve to magnify the vibrations before sending them to the stirrup (stapes) bone. Next, the vibrations pass through the inner ear, i.e., through the scala vestibuli, scala tympani, and cochlea. A fluid called perilymph fills the interior of the cochlea. The vibrations are changed into electric signals in the hair cells in the organ of Corti, which is located on the basilar membrane. The signals are then transmitted via the auditory nerves to the auditory center of the cerebrum to be perceived as sound.

The Vestibular Organs of the Ear. Adjacent to the cochlea in the inner ear are the semicircular ducts, utricle, and saccule. The semicircular ducts include three ducts forming half circles that intersect each other at right angles. When the head is turned a fluid called endolymph inside the semicircular ducts moves, causing the hair cells inside the ampulla of the semicircular ducts to move, which sends signals regarding acceleration or deceleration of rotation to the vestibular nerves.

The utricle and saccule, two membranous organs, contain the maculae. Maculae consist of sensory hair cells and otoliths. When the head is vertical, the utricle is horizontal and the hair cells face up, whereas the saccule is perpendicular and the hair cells face sideways. Gravity and linear acceleration and deceleration to the head are sensed by the change in force perceived by these hair cells.

Adjustment of Air Pressure in the Inner Ear. The inner ear is connected to the pharynx via the auditory tube. When there is a large rapid change in air pressure, which happens in airplanes during landing and takeoff, the semicircular ducts cannot handle the change in air pressure inside and outside the eardrum quickly enough. The eardrum becomes depressed on one side and can no longer respond to the vibration of the air. The pressure inside and outside the eardrum can be equalized by opening the mouth wide or swallowing, which opens the entrance of the auditory tube to the pharynx.

Major Disorders: outer ear infection, middle ear infection (acute, chronic), hearing impairment, Meniere's disease.

2. THE EAR AS AN ORGAN OF HEARING

1. Structure and Pathway of Sound

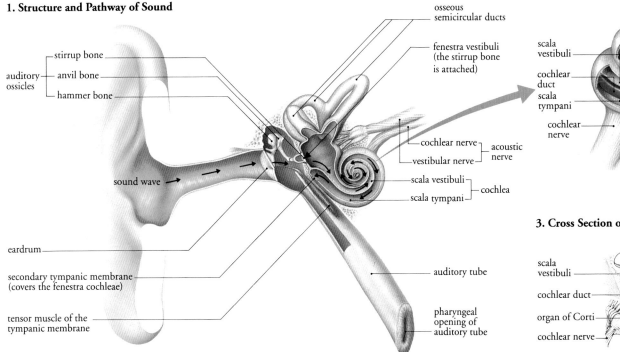

auditory ossicles
- stirrup bone
- anvil bone
- hammer bone

osseous semicircular ducts

fenestra vestibuli (the stirrup bone is attached)

cochlear nerve ┐
vestibular nerve ┘ acoustic nerve

scala vestibuli ┐
scala tympani ┘ cochlea

sound wave

eardrum

secondary tympanic membrane (covers the fenestra cochleae)

tensor muscle of the tympanic membrane

auditory tube

pharyngeal opening of auditory tube

On their way to the inner ear, sound vibrations are transmitted by the eardrum and ear bones to the scala vestibuli, scala tympani and the spiral-shaped cochlea (which is filled with perilymph). Finally, the vibrations are absorbed by the secondary tympanic membrane. In the process, the organ of Corti (Figure 2-2) seizes the vibrations and transforms them into electric signals. These signals are then sent to the cerebrum via the cochlear nerve (auditory nerve). In this figure the cochlear duct has been omitted so the pathway of the sound vibration can be seen.

2. Location of the Cochlear Duct Inside the Cochlea

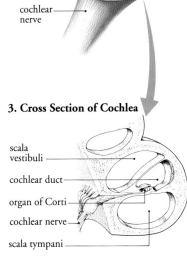

scala vestibuli

cochlear duct

scala tympani

cochlear nerve

3. Cross Section of Cochlea

scala vestibuli

cochlear duct

organ of Corti

cochlear nerve

scala tympani

3. THE EAR AS AN ORGAN OF BALANCE

1. Structure

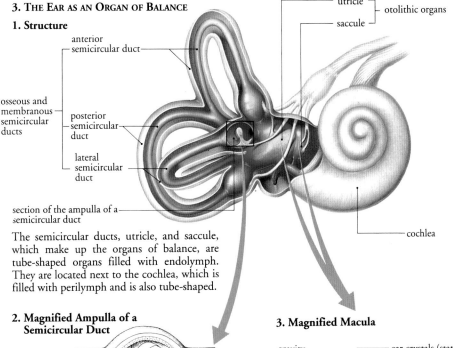

utricle ┐
saccule ┘ otolithic organs

anterior semicircular duct

osseous and membranous semicircular ducts

posterior semicircular duct

lateral semicircular duct

section of the ampulla of a semicircular duct

cochlea

The semicircular ducts, utricle, and saccule, which make up the organs of balance, are tube-shaped organs filled with endolymph. They are located next to the cochlea, which is filled with perilymph and is also tube-shaped.

2. Magnified Ampulla of a Semicircular Duct

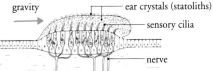

flow of lymph

ampullary crest

nerve

The hair cells of the ampullary crest sense movement, such as rotation of the head, by changes in the flow of endolymph.

3. Magnified Macula

gravity

ear crystals (statoliths)

sensory cilia

nerve

The hair cells sense the direction and linear movements of the body.

4. AUDITORY PATHWAY TO THE CEREBRUM

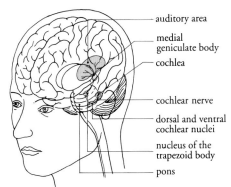

auditory area

medial geniculate body

cochlea

cochlear nerve

dorsal and ventral cochlear nuclei

nucleus of the trapezoid body

pons

This illustration shows the major nerve pathways that sound waves take on their way to the auditory area of the cerebrum.

5. EQUILIBRIAL PATHWAY TO THE CEREBRUM

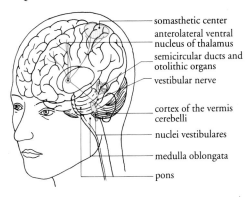

somasthetic center

anterolateral ventral nucleus of thalamus

semicircular ducts and otolithic organs

vestibular nerve

cortex of the vermis cerebelli

nuclei vestibulares

medulla oblongata

pons

The sense of balance as perceived by the semicircular ducts, utricle, and saccule reaches the somesthetic area of the cerebrum mainly via the nerves shown above.

The Nose

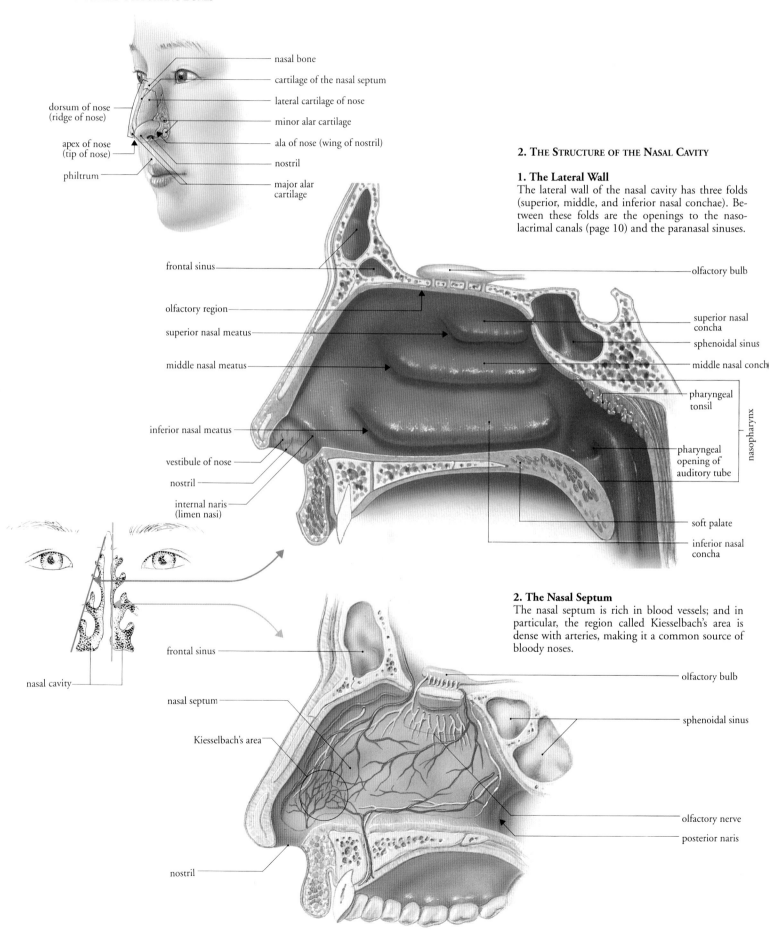

1. The Nose and Supporting Bones

nasal bone

cartilage of the nasal septum

lateral cartilage of nose

minor alar cartilage

ala of nose (wing of nostril)

nostril

major alar cartilage

dorsum of nose (ridge of nose)

apex of nose (tip of nose)

philtrum

2. The Structure of the Nasal Cavity

1. The Lateral Wall
The lateral wall of the nasal cavity has three folds (superior, middle, and inferior nasal conchae). Between these folds are the openings to the naso-lacrimal canals (page 10) and the paranasal sinuses.

frontal sinus

olfactory region

superior nasal meatus

middle nasal meatus

inferior nasal meatus

vestibule of nose

nostril

internal naris (limen nasi)

olfactory bulb

superior nasal concha

sphenoidal sinus

middle nasal conch

pharyngeal tonsil

pharyngeal opening of auditory tube

soft palate

inferior nasal concha

nasopharynx

nasal cavity

2. The Nasal Septum
The nasal septum is rich in blood vessels; and in particular, the region called Kiesselbach's area is dense with arteries, making it a common source of bloody noses.

frontal sinus

nasal septum

Kiesselbach's area

nostril

olfactory bulb

sphenoidal sinus

olfactory nerve

posterior naris

3. PARTS AND LOCATION OF THE PARANASAL SINUSES

1. Anterior View of the Paranasal Sinuses

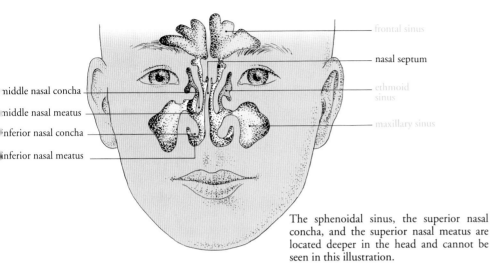

The sphenoidal sinus, the superior nasal concha, and the superior nasal meatus are located deeper in the head and cannot be seen in this illustration.

2. Lateral View of the Paranasal Sinuses

3. Superior View of the Paranasal Sinuses

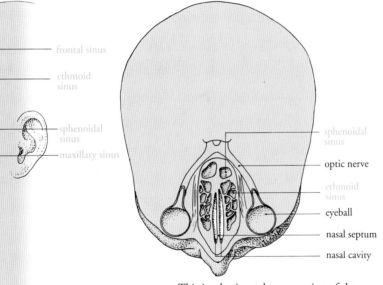

This is a horizontal cross-section of the eyeballs. The frontal sinus, located above the eyeball, and the maxillary sinus, located below the eyeball, cannot be seen.

4. OLFACTORY PATHWAY TO THE CEREBRUM

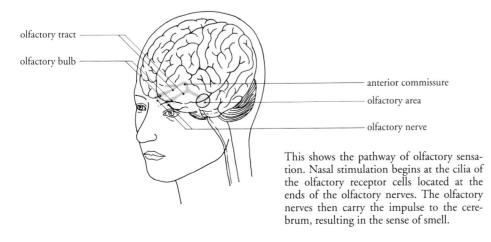

This shows the pathway of olfactory sensation. Nasal stimulation begins at the cilia of the olfactory receptor cells located at the ends of the olfactory nerves. The olfactory nerves then carry the impulse to the cerebrum, resulting in the sense of smell.

The nose functions in the respiratory system as the opening for the passage of air. In addition it is the organ of the sense of smell and is involved in voice production.

Structure. Bone support occurs in the upper half of the nose, whereas most of the lower half, including the wings of the nostrils, is cartilage. The center of the nasal cavity is the nasal septum. Four paranasal sinuses (maxillary, ethmoidal, frontal, and sphenoidal) communicate with the nasal cavity.

The area inside the nares where nasal hair grows is called the vestibule. Farther inside the nasal cavity are the conchae, and beyond these is the nasopharynx (upper pharynx). The nasopharynx is located above the oropharynx, which can be seen when the mouth is open. The soft palate marks the boundary between the nasopharynx and oropharynx.

The nasal conchae are shelflike protrusions on the walls of the nasal cavity. The mucous glands are found on the lowest of these— the inferior nasal concha. On the surface of the conchae are cilia that continuously undulate to move mucus toward the external naris. The uppermost part of the nasal cavity is the region where the olfactory organs are located.

Function. The functions of the nasal cavity include cleaning, heating, and moistening the air as it is breathed in. Inhaled air passes mainly through the middle nasal meatus (above the inferior nasal concha), where 60–70% of the dust is removed and it is converted to a temperature of 25–35°C and a humidity of 35–80%.

Mucous membranes line the nasal cavity. The olfactory receptor cells are located in the superior nasal conchae, and many olfactory cilia are located in the surface mucous membrane. The minute particles that are the source of a smell dissolve in the mucus and stimulate these cilia, which transformss them into electric signals. The signals travel through the olfactory bulb and reach the olfactory center of the cerebral neocortex, resulting in sensory perception of smell.

It is believed that the paranasal sinuses were formed as secondary structures, the result of absorption of parts of bones that had no pressure applied to them and that did not serve any particular purpose. A person's tone or vocal property is formed as the combined result of resonance from the pharynx, oral cavity, and nasal cavity. The nasal cavity is especially involved in forming the sounds of "m," "n," and "g."

Major Disorders: acute rhinitis, chronic rhinitis (simple, hypertrophic, atrophic), allergy, sinusitis, olfactory disorder, curvature of the nasal septum.

The Oral Cavity and Teeth

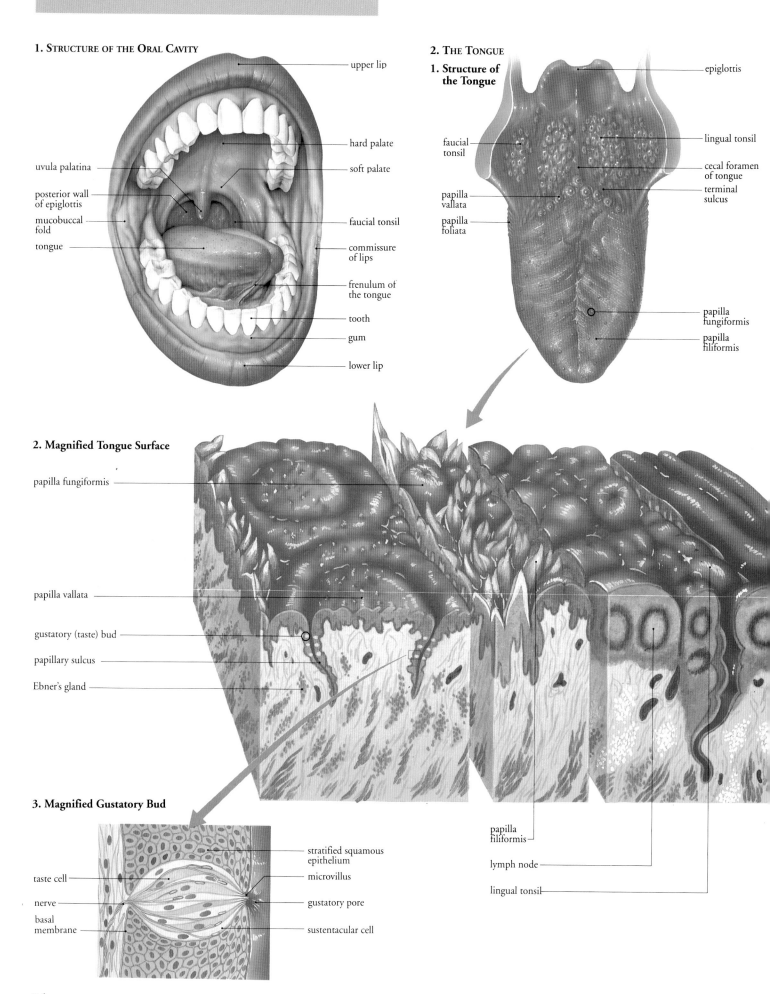

1. STRUCTURE OF THE ORAL CAVITY

upper lip

hard palate

soft palate

uvula palatina

faucial tonsil

posterior wall of epiglottis

mucobuccal fold

commissure of lips

tongue

frenulum of the tongue

tooth

gum

lower lip

2. THE TONGUE

1. Structure of the Tongue

epiglottis

faucial tonsil

lingual tonsil

cecal foramen of tongue

terminal sulcus

papilla vallata

papilla foliata

papilla fungiformis

papilla filiformis

2. Magnified Tongue Surface

papilla fungiformis

papilla vallata

gustatory (taste) bud

papillary sulcus

Ebner's gland

papilla filiformis

lymph node

lingual tonsil

3. Magnified Gustatory Bud

stratified squamous epithelium

microvillus

taste cell

gustatory pore

nerve

basal membrane

sustentacular cell

24

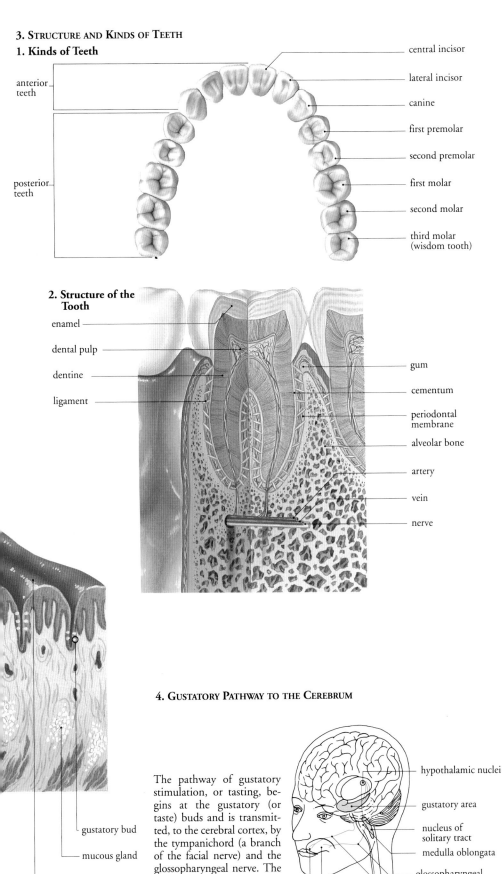

3. Structure and Kinds of Teeth

1. Kinds of Teeth

anterior teeth

posterior teeth

central incisor

lateral incisor

canine

first premolar

second premolar

first molar

second molar

third molar (wisdom tooth)

2. Structure of the Tooth

enamel

dental pulp

dentine

ligament

gum

cementum

periodontal membrane

alveolar bone

artery

vein

nerve

gustatory bud

mucous gland

papilla foliata

4. Gustatory Pathway to the Cerebrum

The pathway of gustatory stimulation, or tasting, begins at the gustatory (or taste) buds and is transmitted, to the cerebral cortex, by the tympanichord (a branch of the facial nerve) and the glossopharyngeal nerve. The tympanichord serves the anterior two-thirds of the tongue and the glossopharyngeal nerve serves the posterior one-third.

hypothalamic nuclei

gustatory area

nucleus of solitary tract

medulla oblongata

glossopharyngeal nerve

tympanichord (branch of facial nerve)

gustatory buds of tongue

The boundaries of the oral cavity include the lips, cheeks, palate, and floor of the mouth. The tongue, with its gustatory organs and teeth for chewing food, are located in the oral cavity.

Structure. The upper part of the oral cavity is the palate, and it separates the oral cavity from the nasal cavity. The anterior two-thirds of the palate is the bony hard palate. The posterior one-third is the soft palate, which is made up of muscle and aponeurosis. Saliva from the parotid gland is secreted into the oral cavity through a duct found at the back of the upper jaw. The tongue is located over the floor of the oral cavity, and the openings of the other salivary glands, the submandibular glands and the sublingual glands, are found here.

Tongue. The tongue is formed by bundles of internal striated muscles running longitudinally and laterally and by external muscles attached to the surrounding bones. The surface is covered with mucous membrane that is dotted with gustatory buds—the receptors of taste. The gustatory buds are concentrated in the anterior two-thirds of the tongue in the fungiform papillae and in the papillae circumvallate, which are found in the posterior part of the tongue. Sweet and salty tastes are sensed toward the tip, acidic taste is sensed at the sides, and bitter taste is sensed at the root of the tongue.

Tonsils. The tonsils are tissues that produce lymphocytes. In the oral cavity, the lingual tonsils are located on both sides at the base of the tongue. The pharyngeal tonsil is located in the posterior wall of the nasopharynx. The palatine tonsils are located in the back of the palate.

Teeth. Deciduous, or primary, teeth begin to grow at about eight months of age, and the set of 20 is complete by about two to three years of age. The 32 permanent teeth replace these between ages six and eleven years.

Function. The tongue and teeth work together to chew food, mix it with saliva, and send it to the pharynx. The oral cavity also works in conjunction with the nasal cavity as a box to amplify the sounds produced by the vocal cords. When swallowing food or voicing sounds, the soft palate moves upward to the rear to touch the posterior wall of the pharynx in order to prevent food and inhaled air from passing into the nasal cavity.

Major Disorders: stomatitis (catarrhal, aphthous, chronic), angular stomatitis, glossitis, gustatory dysgensia, dental caries, pyorrhea.

The Pharynx and Larynx

•**Pharynx:** Length: approx 12–15 cm
•**Larynx:** Length: approx 3–4 cm

1. STRUCTURE OF THE THROAT

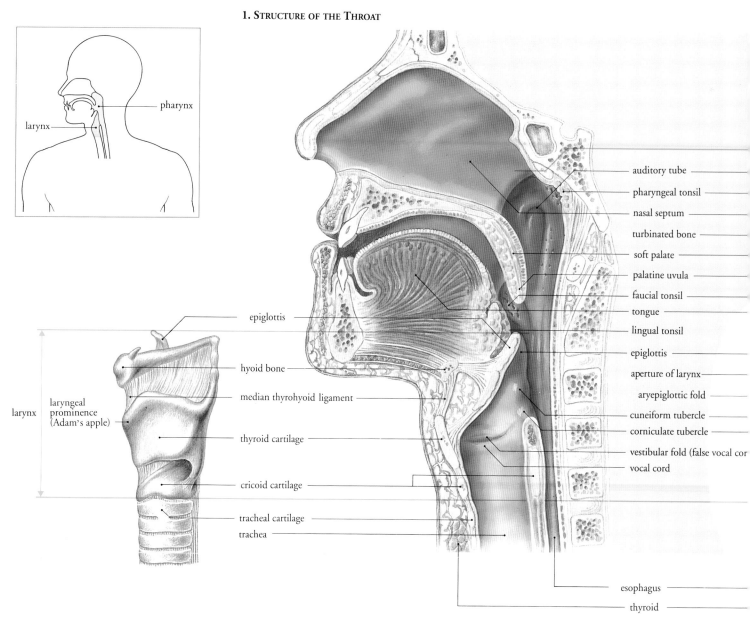

1. Larynx Viewed from the Side
Only the skeletal frame is shown.

2. Section of Throat

The pharynx is the tubal part of the throat that connects the nasal and oral cavities. The larynx, branching off from the pharynx, is the air passageway communicating with the trachea. In the adult male, the cartilage that surrounds the larynx and protrudes from the front of the neck is called the "Adam's apple."

THE PHARYNX

Structure. The opening of the pharynx is visible when the mouth is open. It is approx 12–15 cm in length and runs parallel to the spinal column, forming a cylinder that is flat on the front and back. The upper end is a dome (vault of the pharynx), touching the base of the skull, and the lower end joins the esophagus. The anterior of the pharynx is connected to the nasal cavity and the oral cavity between the soft palate and root of the tongue. The pharynx communicates with the larynx at the epiglottis. The wall of the pharynx is composed of layers of striated muscle.

Function. The pharynx is the intersection between the air passage (the nasal cavity, pharynx, larynx, and trachea) and the food passage the oral cavity, pharynx, and esophagus. The epiglottis plays the important role of preventing food from entering the air passageway.

THE LARYNX

Structure. The thyroid cartilage, the cricoid cartilage, and the epiglottis form a framework, inside which are located numerous additional cartilage muscles and vocal cords. Mucous membrane lines the inner wall of the larynx and covers the cartilage and mus-

2. STRUCTURE OF THE VOCAL CORDS

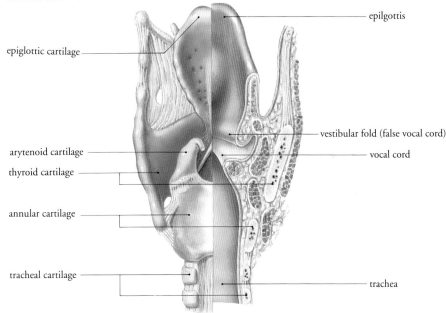

epilgottis

epiglottic cartilage

vestibular fold (false vocal cord)

vocal cord

arytenoid cartilage

thyroid cartilage

annular cartilage

tracheal cartilage

trachea

Pharynx, viewed from the rear. Left half shows only the skeletal structure while the right side is a vertical section.

3. THE VOCAL CORDS AS SEEN IN A MIRROR FROM ABOVE

1. How the Mirror is Placed for Observation

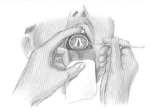

2. The Vocal Cords Between Breaths

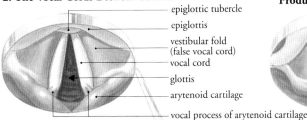

epiglottic tubercle

epiglottis

vestibular fold (false vocal cord)

vocal cord

glottis

arytenoid cartilage

vocal process of arytenoid cartilage

3. The Vocal Cords When a Deep Breath is Being Taken

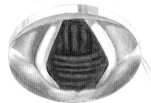

4. The Vocal Cords When Producing Sound

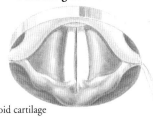

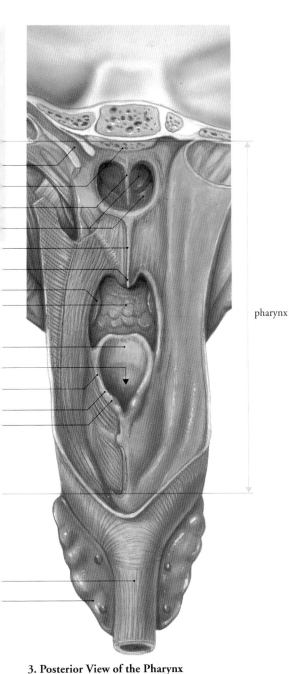

pharynx

3. Posterior View of the Pharynx
The mucous membrane has been omitted on the left side to show the muscles.

4. HOW THE SOFT PALATE AND EPIGLOTTIS WORK TO AVOID CONFUSION

1. Breathing

2. Swallowing

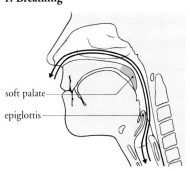
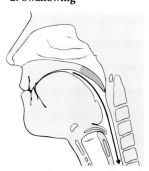

soft palate

epiglottis

When breathing, the soft palate and epiglottis open the trachea reflexively. When swallowing food, the soft palate moves to the rear to open the esophagus and prevent backflow to the nose and auditory tubes, while the epiglottis closes off the air passage to prevent food and other matter from entering the trachea.

cles. At the center of the larynx, two folds of mucous membrane form the false vocal cords and the vocal cords.

Function. The larynx is the boundary between the upper air passageway and the lower air passageway. Its width adjusts to control breathing and to protect the passage. The vocal cords produce sounds for speech. The epiglottis opens when inhaling and narrows when exhaling. When swallowing food or vomiting, the epiglottis, false vocal cords, and vocal cords close the laryngeal cavity, preventing foreign matter from entering the larynx from the pharynx.

Major Disorders: facial tonsillitis, pharyngitis, adenoids, cancer of the upper jaw, laryngitis, polyps of the vocal cords.

2 *The Thorax*

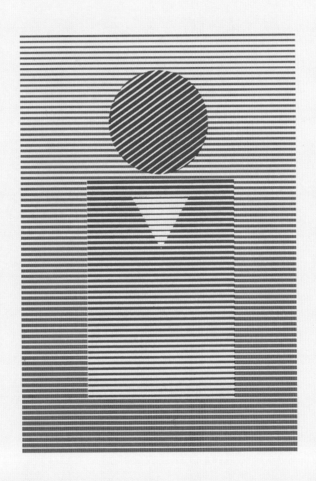

The Thorax

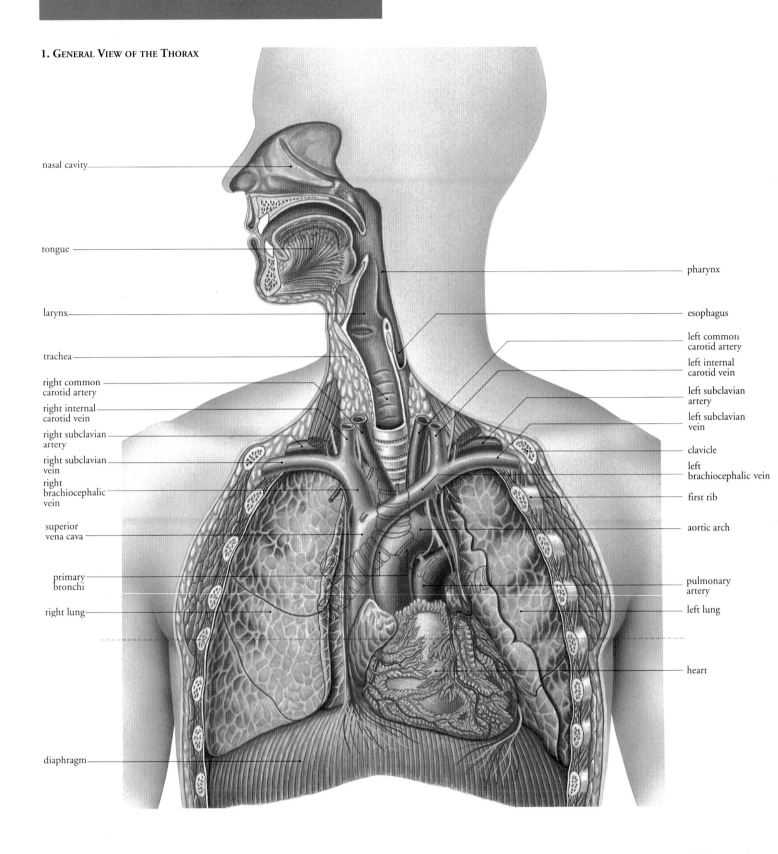

nasal cavity

tongue

larynx

trachea

right common carotid artery

right internal carotid vein

right subclavian artery

right subclavian vein

right brachiocephalic vein

superior vena cava

primary bronchi

right lung

diaphragm

pharynx

esophagus

left common carotid artery

left internal carotid vein

left subclavian artery

left subclavian vein

clavicle

left brachiocephalic vein

first rib

aortic arch

pulmonary artery

left lung

heart

The area below the neck from the shoulders to the 12th thoracic vertebra is known as the thorax (chest). On the ventral side the boundary between the thorax and the abdomen is the lower end of the sternum (breastbone).

The skeletal part of the thorax forms a cage of bones and muscles that protects the heart and lungs, the organs of circulation and respiration. The sternum is a long narrow bone made up of three parts: the manubrium, the body, and the xiphoid process.

The sternum, together with the 12 thoracic vertebrae of the spinal column, form vertical supports in the front and back. These supports are connected by 12 pairs of ribs and costal cartilage, forming the rib cage.

Viewed from the front, part of the heart is visible between the left and right lung. Viewed from the side, the lung is spread out and covers the heart and spinal column (Figure 2).

A horizontal cross-secton of the thorax at the nipples reveals the

2. Organs of the Thorax and Protective Skeletal Framework

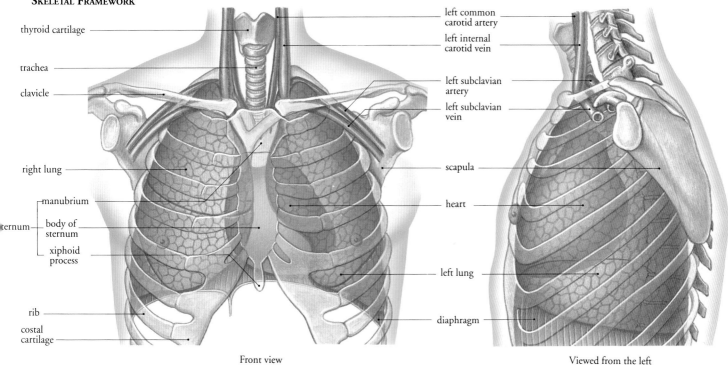

thyroid cartilage

trachea

clavicle

right lung

manubrium

body of sternum

xiphoid process

sternum

rib

costal cartilage

left common carotid artery

left internal carotid vein

left subclavian artery

left subclavian vein

scapula

heart

left lung

diaphragm

Front view

Viewed from the left

3. Cross Section of the Thorax

Dorsum

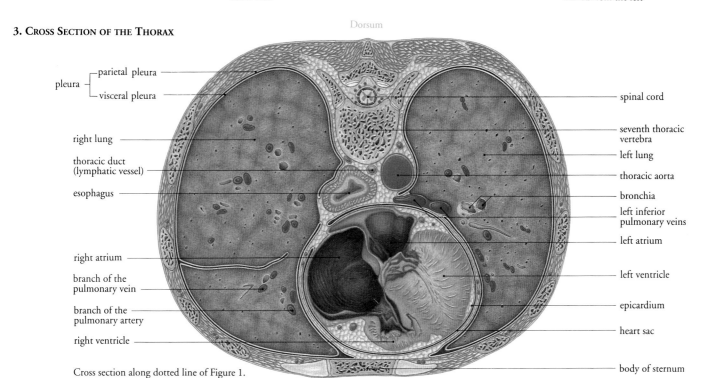

pleura

parietal pleura

visceral pleura

right lung

thoracic duct (lymphatic vessel)

esophagus

right atrium

branch of the pulmonary vein

branch of the pulmonary artery

right ventricle

spinal cord

seventh thoracic vertebra

left lung

thoracic aorta

bronchia

left inferior pulmonary veins

left atrium

left ventricle

epicardium

heart sac

body of sternum

Cross section along dotted line of Figure 1.

thoracic aorta and the star-shaped section of the esophagus situated between the thoracic vertebrae (spinal column) and the heart and lungs (Figure 3).

The space bordered by the sternum, the thoracic vertebrae, and the lungs is known as the mediastinum. It houses the thick arteries and veins entering and exiting the heart and lungs, as well as the trachea, esophagus, lymph vessels, and nerves to the neck. Just behind the sternum is the thymus gland, a part of the endocrine system.

The opening to the thorax at the neck is bordered by the first rib, the first thoracic vertebra, and the manubrium. The trachea and esophagus as well as nerves and blood vessels enter and exit the thorax here. Across the thoracic opening a "cape" of muscles stretches among the collar bones, shoulder bones, and upper arm bones. These muscles work with the muscles between the upper arms and ribs to move the upper limbs.

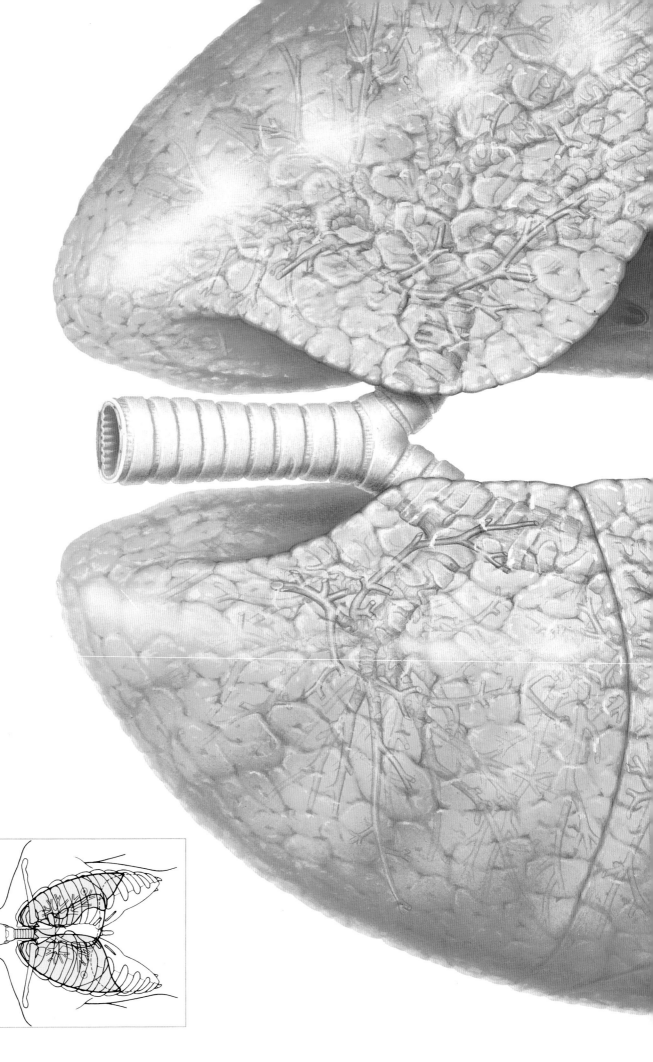

The Lungs, Trachea, and Bronchus

- **Lungs:** Weight: males, approx 1060 g; females, approx 930 g
- **Trachea:** Length: approx 10–11 cm, width left-to-right: approx 1.5 cm
- **Bronchi:** Length: left primary bronchus, approx 4–6 cm; right primary bronchus, approx 3 cm

1. LUNG SHOWN ACTUAL SIZE

2. BIFURCATION OF THE TRACHEA AND NAMES OF THE PARTS BEYOND

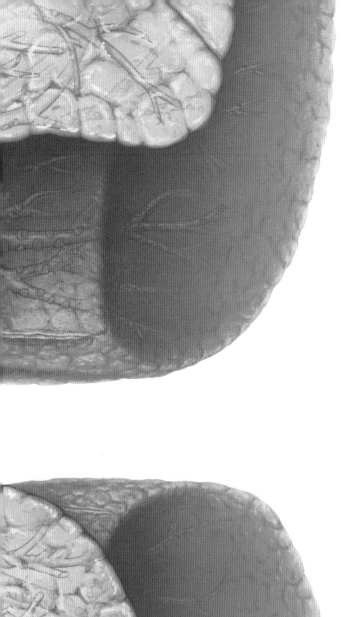

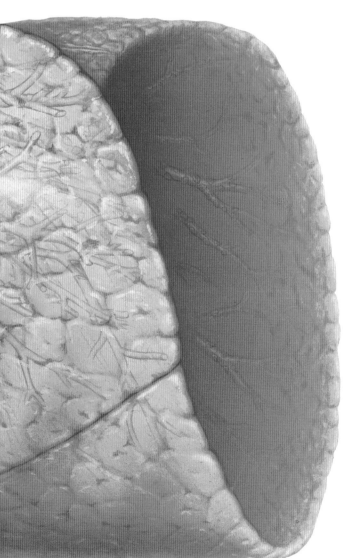

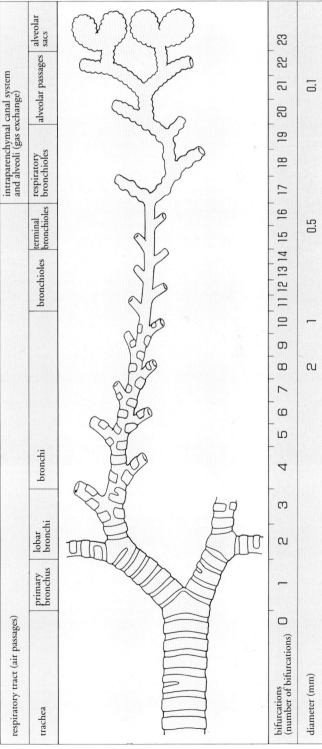

respiratory tract (air passages)							intraparenchymal canal system and alveoli (gas exchange)		
trachea	primary bronchus	lobar bronchi	bronchi	bronchioles	terminal bronchioles	respiratory bronchioles	alveolar passages	alveolar sacs
bifurcations (number of bifurcations) 0 1 2 3 4 5 6 7 8 9 10 11 12 13 14 15 16 17 18 19 20 21 22 23
diameter (mm) 2   1   0.5   0.1

The trachea branches into the left and right primary bronchi at the fourth and fifth thoracic vertebrae. The bronchi further branch at irregular intervals, narrowing gradually until they reach the bronchioles and, finally, the alveoli, where gases are exchanged. There is no cartilage beyond the bronchiole. The number of times the bronchi branch before reaching the bronchiole varies from lung to lung. Here we show the average number of branches (16).

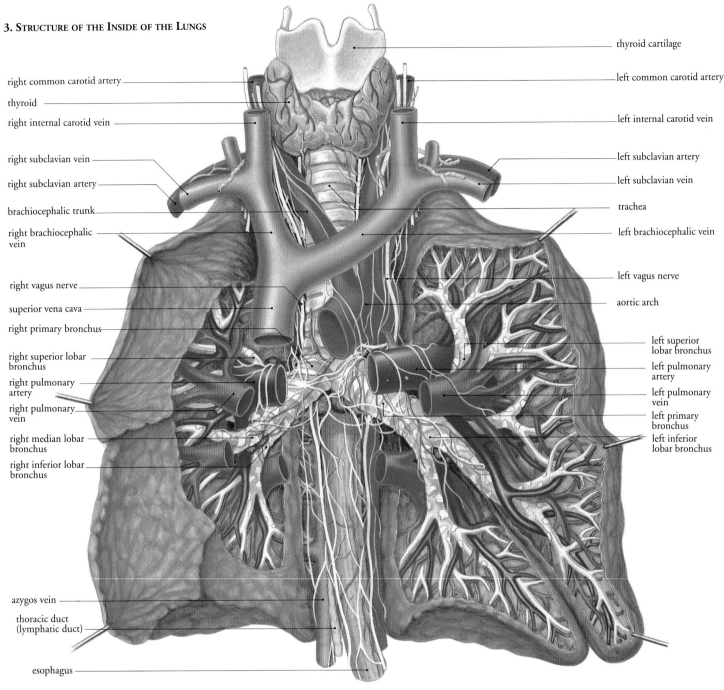

right common carotid artery

thyroid

right internal carotid vein

right subclavian vein

right subclavian artery

brachiocephalic trunk

right brachiocephalic vein

right vagus nerve

superior vena cava

right primary bronchus

right superior lobar bronchus

right pulmonary artery

right pulmonary vein

right median lobar bronchus

right inferior lobar bronchus

azygos vein

thoracic duct (lymphatic duct)

esophagus

thyroid cartilage

left common carotid artery

left internal carotid vein

left subclavian artery

left subclavian vein

trachea

left brachiocephalic vein

left vagus nerve

aortic arch

left superior lobar bronchus

left pulmonary artery

left pulmonary vein

left primary bronchus

left inferior lobar bronchus

Interior of the lungs with the heart removed.

In the lung, venous blood from the heart is infused with fresh oxygen and carbon dioxide is removed, in a process called gas exchange. The trachea, or windpipe, and bronchi are the passages for the gases.

LUNG

Location and Size. The lungs are the largest organs located inside the thorax. Males: average approx 1060 g (right lung approx 570 g, left lung approx 490 g). Females: average approx 930 g (right lung approx 500 g, left lung approx 430 g).

Function. The lungs exchange carbon dioxide for oxygenated blood.

Structure. The pulmonary arteries leading from the right ventricle of the heart transport blood to the lungs, whereas the bronchi and bronchioles transport air. A significant part of the lung is occupied by these two types of passages (Figure 3). The pulmonary arteries (through which venous blood flows) follow the bifurcations of the bronchi and become capillaries. After irrigating the walls of the alveoli, they become veins (through which arterial blood flows) and return to the left atrium of the heart.

The lung is divided into sections, or lobes, by fissures. The right lung is divided into three parts: the upper, middle, and lower lobes; and the left lung is divided into two parts: the upper and lower lobes (Figure 4-1). These lobes are further divided into smaller regions.

TRACHEA

The trachea is a pipe approx 10–11 cm long and 1.5 cm in diameter, which leads from the juncture of the larynx in the neck re-

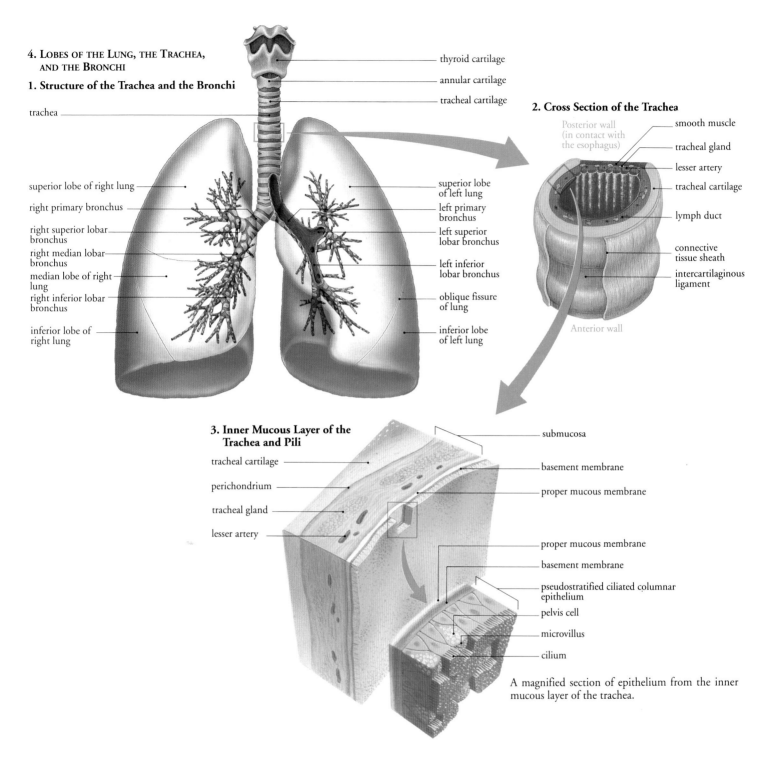

4. Lobes of the Lung, the Trachea, and the Bronchi

1. Structure of the Trachea and the Bronchi

trachea

thyroid cartilage

annular cartilage

tracheal cartilage

superior lobe of right lung

right primary bronchus

right superior lobar bronchus

right median lobar bronchus

median lobe of right lung

right inferior lobar bronchus

inferior lobe of right lung

superior lobe of left lung

left primary bronchus

left superior lobar bronchus

left inferior lobar bronchus

oblique fissure of lung

inferior lobe of left lung

2. Cross Section of the Trachea

Posterior wall (in contact with the esophagus)

smooth muscle

tracheal gland

lesser artery

tracheal cartilage

lymph duct

connective tissue sheath

intercartilaginous ligament

Anterior wall

3. Inner Mucous Layer of the Trachea and Pili

tracheal cartilage

perichondrium

tracheal gland

lesser artery

submucosa

basement membrane

proper mucous membrane

proper mucous membrane

basement membrane

pseudostratified ciliated columnar epithelium

pelvis cell

microvillus

cilium

A magnified section of epithelium from the inner mucous layer of the trachea.

gion to the point of bifurcation into the bronchi. To reinforce the trachea 10–20 tracheal cartilages shaped like horseshoes are found attached around the front and sides. The posterior wall of the trachea, where there is no cartilage, is covered by membranous tissue, and the inner side of the entire trachea is lined with mucous membrane. The surface of the mucous membrane is covered by a ciliated epithelium and the proper mucous membrane of the inner side is very elastic. Tracheal glands that secrete mucus are distributed throughout the submucous (Figure 4-3). Cilia move ceaselessly in a wavelike motion toward the direction of the mouth, capturing particles of dust and other invading matter so they can be expelled with mucous.

BRONCHI

The trachea branches into two primary bronchi, one entering

the left lung and the other entering the right lung. The left primary bronchus is approx 4–6 cm in length and is longer than the right primary bronchus, which is approx 3 cm in length. The primary bronchi continue to bifurcate and, at the 17th–19th bifurcation, they eventually terminate at the bronchioles (diameter approx 0.5 mm). Beyond the respiratory bronchiole are the alveoli. The bronchi of the lungs are like a tree: The bronchioles leading to and from the alveoli are like the branches and stems and the alveoli correspond to the leaves (see page 33, Figure 2).

Major Disorders: lung cancer, pneumonia, pulmonary edema, pulmonary cysts, pulmonary tuberculosis, bronchial asthma, bronchitis, bronchial obstruction, bronchiectasis.

The Alveoli and Gas Exchange

ALVEOLI

Round alveoli protrude like berries from the alveolar ducts, which in turn descend from the bronchioles and the bronchi. In the adult, alveolar ducts number approx 14 million, and each duct has an average of 20 alveoli, bringing the total number of alveoli for both lungs to approx 600 million. Each alveolus is approx 0.14 mm in diameter. The area of alveoli involved in gas exchange is approx 60 mm, and about 75% of the alveolar wall surface area is covered by a network of capillaries.

GAS EXCHANGE

During normal respiration, approx 2500 ml of air remains in the lungs after exhalation (functional residual capacity). As a result, pure fresh air does not enter the alveoli for gas exchange. After inhaling fresh air, the concentration of oxygen (partial pressure of oxygen) in the air that enters the alveoli is diluted by some of the residual air. The oxygen in the alveoli and the carbon dioxide in the red corpuscles pass through a membrane 0.001 mm thick; the membrane is comprised of the walls of both the alveolus and the capillary. The gas with higher partial pressure takes the place of the gas with lower partial pressure, resulting in gas exchange.

RESPIRATION AND CIRCULATION

Respiration and circulation are closely intertwined. For example, to resuscitate an individual whose heart and breathing have stopped, artificial respiration and heart massage are necessary. Artificial respiration sends fresh air to the lungs and heart massage circulates blood so gas exchange can take place. This is the way oxygen is supplied to the blood and circulated to the brain and all the other organs. In cardiac asthma, breathing is labored, as in bronchial asthma, and pulmonary circulation is decreased, resulting in oxygen deficiency.

1. GENERAL VIEW OF THE ORGANS OF THE RESPIRATORY TRACT

1. Respiration and Pulmonary Circulation

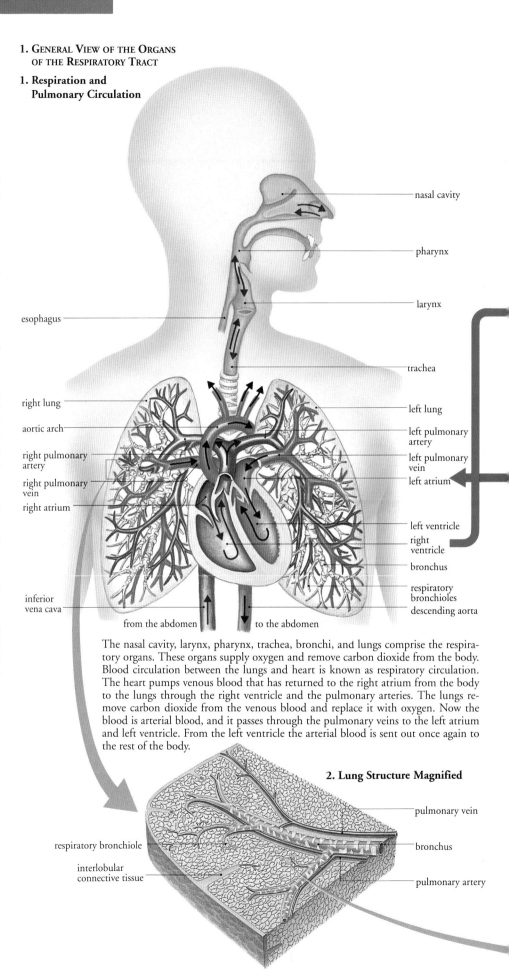

The nasal cavity, larynx, pharynx, trachea, bronchi, and lungs comprise the respiratory organs. These organs supply oxygen and remove carbon dioxide from the body. Blood circulation between the lungs and heart is known as respiratory circulation. The heart pumps venous blood that has returned to the right atrium from the body to the lungs through the right ventricle and the pulmonary arteries. The lungs remove carbon dioxide from the venous blood and replace it with oxygen. Now the blood is arterial blood, and it passes through the pulmonary veins to the left atrium and left ventricle. From the left ventricle the arterial blood is sent out once again to the rest of the body.

2. Lung Structure Magnified

2. ALVEOLI AND GAS EXCHANGE

An alveolus is a sac-shaped tissue (diameter of approx 0.14 mm) with a surface that is covered by a network of capillaries. Gas exchange occurs through the walls of the alveolus and capillary. Venous blood coming from the right ventricle of the heart to the lungs via the pulmonary arteries is changed to arterial blood through this exchange of gases. The blood then returns via the pulmonary vein to the left atrium.

1. Alveoli and Alveolar Capillaries

3. Sample Mold of Alveolar Capillaries

2. How Gas Exchange Occurs

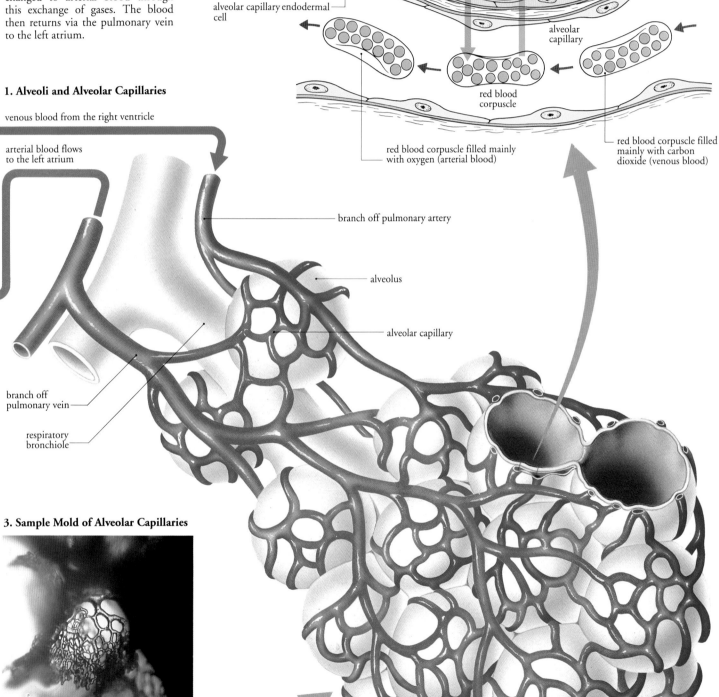

venous blood from the right ventricle

arterial blood flows to the left atrium

branch off pulmonary artery

alveolus

alveolar capillary

branch off pulmonary vein

respiratory bronchiole

surfactant layer

alveolar epidermal cell

alveolar basement membrane

interstitial space

capillary basement membrane

alveolar capillary endodermal cell

carbon dioxide

oxygen

alveolar space

alveolar capillary

red blood corpuscle

red blood corpuscle filled mainly with oxygen (arterial blood)

red blood corpuscle filled mainly with carbon dioxide (venous blood)

Muscles Related to Respiration

1. RESPIRATORY MUSCLES

2. EXPANSION AND CONTRACTION OF THE THORAX AND RESPIRATION

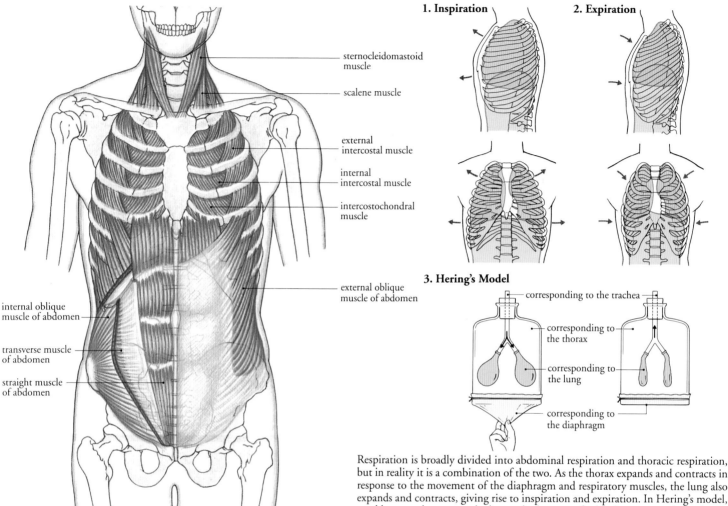

1. Inspiration

2. Expiration

3. Hering's Model

sternocleidomastoid muscle

scalene muscle

external intercostal muscle

internal intercostal muscle

intercostochondral muscle

external oblique muscle of abdomen

internal oblique muscle of abdomen

transverse muscle of abdomen

straight muscle of abdomen

corresponding to the trachea

corresponding to the thorax

corresponding to the lung

corresponding to the diaphragm

Respiration is broadly divided into abdominal respiration and thoracic respiration, but in reality it is a combination of the two. As the thorax expands and contracts in response to the movement of the diaphragm and respiratory muscles, the lung also expands and contracts, giving rise to inspiration and expiration. In Hering's model, a rubber membrane stretched over the bottom of a bottle corresponds to the diaphragm. When this membrane is pulled downward, the internal pressure of the bottle, which corresponds to the thorax, decreases, resulting in the influx of air. The air enters rubber balloons, which correspond to the lungs, and inflates them (inspiration). When the membrane is returned to its original position, the internal pressure rises, deflating the balloons (expiration).

Respiration does not occur solely as a result of the lungs inflating and deflating under their own power. It occurs as a result of expansion and contraction of the thorax enclosing the lungs, i.e., the diaphragm and intercostal muscles.

THE DIAPHRAGM

Hering's model (Figure 2-3) is used to explain how respiration occurs. The bottle used in this model corresponds to the thorax, which is made of bones and muscles, and the rubber membrane stretched across the bottom of the bottle corresponds to the diaphragm. The lung and the bronchi in the lung are lined with thoracic membrane so there is no leakage of air. The pipe that extends outside the bottle corresponds to the trachea. If the rubber membrane of the model is pulled downward, the pressure inside the bottle decreases, and air enters the rubber balloons and inflates them. Like the model, when the thorax expands, because of the operation of the diaphragm and intercostal muscles, the pressure inside the thorax decreases, letting in air from the trachea and expanding the highly flexible lungs. When the thorax contracts, the lungs are compressed and air is expelled from the lungs. When relaxed, the di-

aphragm is in the shape of an upside-down pan. When the muscles of the diaphragm contract, the bottom of the diaphragm becomes flat and sinks. The change in level is as much as 7–10 cm. When the muscles relax, the capacity of the thorax returns to normal and air from the lungs is released. Respiration resulting from the function of the diaphragm is known as abdominal respiration. This type of respiration accounts for about 70% of respiration when the body is at rest.

INTERCOSTAL MUSCLES

Intercostal muscles are also involved in the expansion and contraction of the thorax. The external intercostal muscles connect the ribs, and when they contract, the thorax expands and inhalation occurs. When the internal muscles between the ribs contract, the ribs are lowered and the thorax contracts and exhalation occurs. This type of respiration is called thoracic respiration. The muscles of the thoracic wall, the scalene, and sternocleidomastoid muscles of the neck are also involved in thoracic respiration. If there is a hole in the thorax or the lungs, no matter how hard the respiratory muscles work, the pressure inside and outside remains the same, making it impossible for the lungs to inflate and respiration to occur.

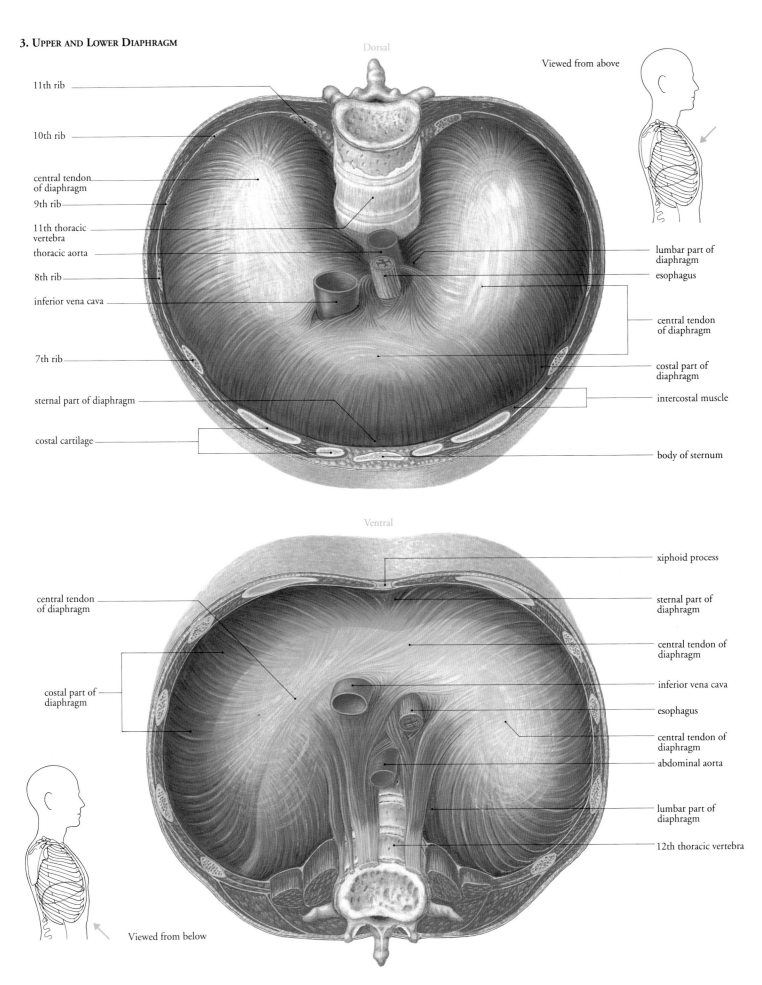

Dorsal

Viewed from above

11th rib

10th rib

central tendon
of diaphragm

9th rib

11th thoracic
vertebra

thoracic aorta

8th rib

inferior vena cava

7th rib

sternal part of diaphragm

costal cartilage

lumbar part of
diaphragm

esophagus

central tendon
of diaphragm

costal part of
diaphragm

intercostal muscle

body of sternum

Ventral

central tendon
of diaphragm

costal part of
diaphragm

Viewed from below

xiphoid process

sternal part of
diaphragm

central tendon of
diaphragm

inferior vena cava

esophagus

central tendon of
diaphragm

abdominal aorta

lumbar part of
diaphragm

12th thoracic vertebra

39

The Heart

- Length: approx 14 cm, width: approx 10 cm,
- Depth: approx 8 cm, weight: approx 250-300 g

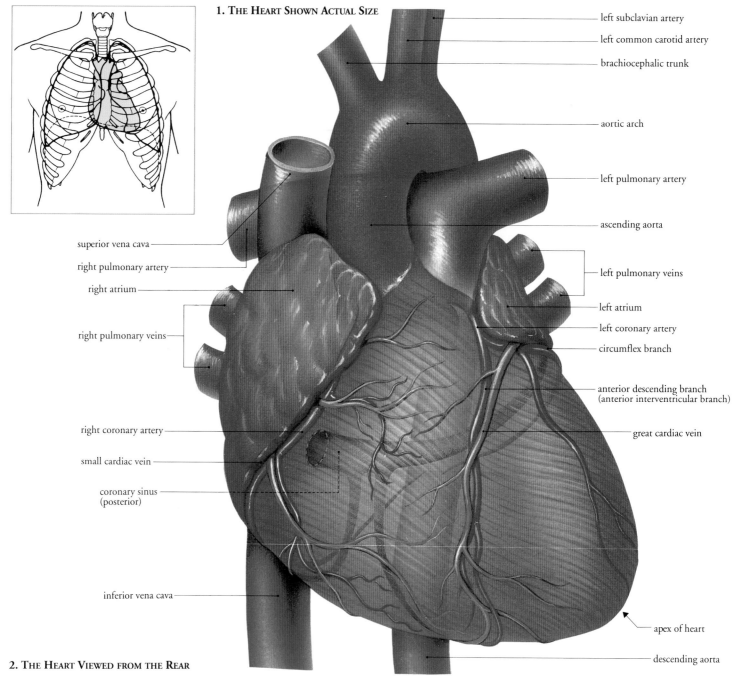

1. THE HEART SHOWN ACTUAL SIZE

- left subclavian artery
- left common carotid artery
- brachiocephalic trunk
- aortic arch
- left pulmonary artery
- ascending aorta
- left pulmonary veins
- left atrium
- left coronary artery
- circumflex branch
- anterior descending branch (anterior interventricular branch)
- great cardiac vein
- apex of heart
- descending aorta

- superior vena cava
- right pulmonary artery
- right atrium
- right pulmonary veins
- right coronary artery
- small cardiac vein
- coronary sinus (posterior)
- inferior vena cava

2. THE HEART VIEWED FROM THE REAR

- left subclavian artery
- left common carotid artery
- left pulmonary artery
- left pulmonary veins
- left atrium
- left ventricle
- brachiocephalic trunk
- aortic arch
- superior vena cava
- right pulmonary artery
- right pulmonary veins
- right atrium
- inferior vena cava

The heart is the organ that pumps blood throughout the body to maintain life. Heart failure was once the main criterion in determining death, but with the development of various life support systems, heart function is no longer the sole criterion. The newer concept of brain death is also considered.

Location. The heart is situated slightly to the left of the center of the thorax, touching the left and right lungs. A cross section through the seventh thoracic vertebra shows that the heart lies almost exactly midway between the spinal column and the sternum. The longitudinal axis of the heart is at approx a 50° angle to the horizontal plane. The bottom edge (apex of heart) is inclined diagonally toward the front, and each time the heart contracts, it hits the inner surface of the thoracic wall.

Size and Shape. The heart is a little larger than the fist. In the adult human, it weighs approx 250–350 g. The atria and ventricles are in the classic "heart" shape, and it also looks like a large peach hanging from branches made up of the large blood vessels.

3. Structure of the Interior of the Heart

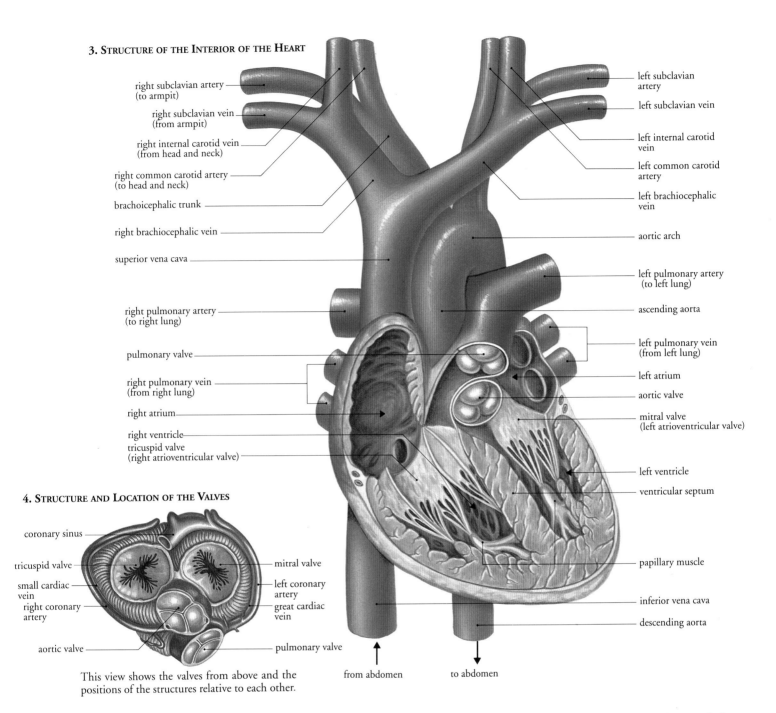

right subclavian artery
(to armpit)

right subclavian vein
(from armpit)

right internal carotid vein
(from head and neck)

right common carotid artery
(to head and neck)

brachoicephalic trunk

right brachiocephalic vein

superior vena cava

right pulmonary artery
(to right lung)

pulmonary valve

right pulmonary vein
(from right lung)

right atrium

right ventricle

tricuspid valve
(right atrioventricular valve)

left subclavian
artery

left subclavian vein

left internal carotid
vein

left common carotid
artery

left brachiocephalic
vein

aortic arch

left pulmonary artery
(to left lung)

ascending aorta

left pulmonary vein
(from left lung)

left atrium

aortic valve

mitral valve
(left atrioventricular valve)

left ventricle

ventricular septum

papillary muscle

inferior vena cava

descending aorta

from abdomen

to abdomen

4. Structure and Location of the Valves

coronary sinus

tricuspid valve

small cardiac
vein

right coronary
artery

aortic valve

mitral valve

left coronary
artery

great cardiac
vein

pulmonary valve

This view shows the valves from above and the
positions of the structures relative to each other.

Structure. The heart is a muscle (cardiac muscle) that contracts and relaxes regularly to pump blood through the body. The inner surface is called the endocardium, and the outermost layer is the epicardium. The interior is divided into four chambers, left and right atria and left and right ventricles.

The heart has four valves, which ensure that blood does not flow in the wrong direction. The valve between the left atrium and left vertricle is the mitral valve and the valve between the right atrium and right ventricle is the tricuspid valve. A ligament extending from the papillary muscle of the ventricles is attached to the rim of the valves to prevent the tip of the valves from bending backward. The pulmonary valve at the opening of the pulmonary artery and the aortic valve at the opening of the aorta are semilunar valves. Semilunar valves are so-called because they are shaped like three half-moons. In the heart, the coronary arteries and veins supply oxygen and energy to the cardiac muscle to maintain its activity. The large blood vessels—aorta, vena cava, pulmonary arteries, and pulmonary veins—transport blood in and out of the heart, allowing it to carry out its function as a pump.

Function. The heart pumps arterial blood, which is rich in oxygen and energy, throughout the body. Blood on its way back to the heart has increased levels of carbon dioxide and waste, which are by-products of energy consumption by the various tissues. This blood is called venous blood. Blood takes on additional energy resources, hormones, and neurotransmitters from the portal system (see page 65), before returning to the right atrium of the heart. The blood is then pumped to the lungs where it releases excess carbon dioxide and takes on fresh oxygen, after which it returns to the heart once more (left atrium) before it is pumped out again through the aorta as arterial blood. The amount of blood pumped in one contraction (stroke volume) varies by body build, but the heart of a person 160 cm tall and weighing 50 kg pumps approx 70 ml, making the output per minute about 5 l.

Blood Vessels Supplying the Heart

1. NETWORK OF CORONARY ARTERIES AND VEINS

1. Anterior Network

2. Posterior Network

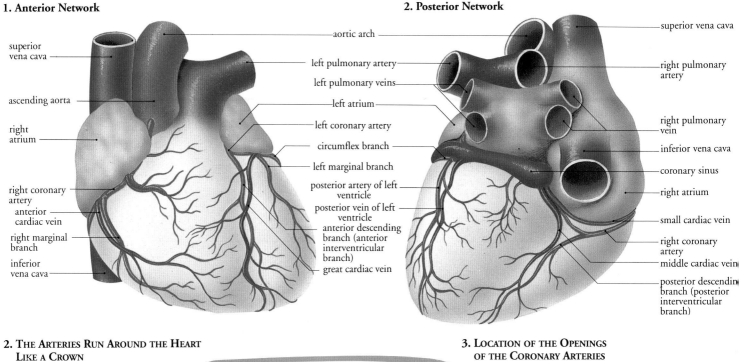

superior vena cava
ascending aorta
right atrium
right coronary artery
anterior cardiac vein
right marginal branch
inferior vena cava

aortic arch
left pulmonary artery
left pulmonary veins
left atrium
left coronary artery
circumflex branch
left marginal branch
posterior artery of left ventricle
posterior vein of left ventricle
anterior descending branch (anterior interventricular branch)
great cardiac vein

superior vena cava
right pulmonary artery
right pulmonary vein
inferior vena cava
coronary sinus
right atrium
small cardiac vein
right coronary artery
middle cardiac vein
posterior descending branch (posterior interventricular branch)

2. THE ARTERIES RUN AROUND THE HEART LIKE A CROWN

superior vena cava
aortic valve
right atrium
right coronary artery
posterior descending branch (posterior interventricular branch)
right marginal branch
inferior vena cava

pulmonary valve
left pulmonary veins
left atrium
circumflex branch
left coronary artery
anterior descending branch (anterior interventricular branch)

The narrow branches have been omitted from this illustration to show how the main branches of the left and right coronary arteries circle the heart like a crown, or corona, which explains why they are called "coronary" arteries.

3. LOCATION OF THE OPENINGS OF THE CORONARY ARTERIES

left coronary artery opening
left semilunar valve
ascending aorta
right coronary artery opening
right semilunar valve
posterior semilunar valve

The left and right openings to the coronary arteries (where the arteries begin) are located near the aortic valve. This illustration shows the aortic valve as viewed diagonally from above left.

Coronary Arteries. The heart is the muscle that pumps out blood throughout the body, but to function, the heart requires its own supply of blood. It would appear that the heart could freely take rich arterial blood for itself. However, like the bank teller who handles large amounts of cash (but is not free to spend it), the life-giving heart is only able to use for itself the blood supplied by the narrow coronary arteries that serve only the heart.

Volume of Blood Required to Supply the Heart. When the body is at rest, approx 80 ml per minute per 100 g of cardiac muscle travels through the left ventricle. Approximately 70–80% of that amount flows through the right ventricle, and about half that volume supplies the left and right atria. Thus approx 250 ml of blood per minute is required for the heart to maintain activity. Because the heart pumps approx 5000 ml of blood per minute, this amounts to about 5% of the volume pumped.

The heart, which works without rest, consumes approx 70% of the oxygen provided by the coronary arteries (the internal organs of the abdominal region consume 15–20%). As a result, the concentration of oxygen in the venous blood of the coronary veins is extremely low—the lowest concentration of all the other tissues and organs.

Because the heart works so hard and uses so much oxygen, it is especially susceptible to oxygen deficiency. If a branch of the coronary arteries becomes obstructed, the tissue around the blood vessel dies (necrosis). This is known as myocardial infarction, and it is feared as one of the primary causes of death.

Pathway of Coronary Circulation. The openings to the left and right coronary arteries (where the arteries begin) are in Valsalva's sinus (aortic sinus) very near the aortic valve at the base of the aorta where it extends from the heart (left ventricle). In keeping with their name, the coronary arteries wrap around the surface of the heart like a crown (under the epicardium) from the

4. How Arteriosclerosis Develops and Lesions of the Coronary Artery

1. Development of Arteriosclerosis

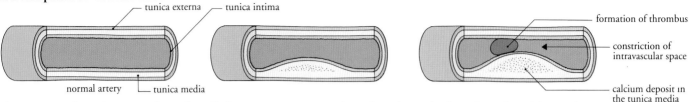

tunica externa — tunica intima

normal artery — tunica media

formation of thrombus

constriction of intravascular space

calcium deposit in the tunica media

The externa, media, and intima make up the wall of an artery. If cholesterol or calcium builds up in the intima or media, the wall becomes thicker, narrowing the intravascular space where blood flows. One of these conditions is known as atherosclerosis. When atherosclerosis develops, the surface of the vessel becomes rough, and this roughness causes blood to clot. The clotted blood now narrows or blocks (thrombosis) the intravascular space, preventing circulation.

2. Lesions of the Coronary Artery

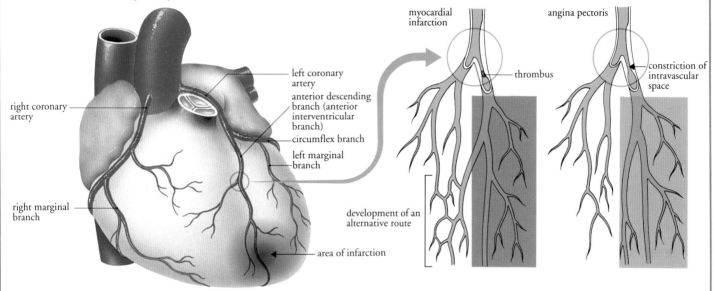

left coronary artery

anterior descending branch (anterior interventricular branch)

circumflex branch

left marginal branch

right coronary artery

right marginal branch

area of infarction

myocardial infarction

angina pectoris

thrombus

constriction of intravascular space

development of an alternative route

Myocardial Infarction. This is a condition in which an obstruction, such as a blood clot, blocks part of a coronary artery, suddenly stopping circulation and causing cardiac muscle tissue to die. This occurs most often in the arteries numbered 1–4 in the illustration above. The numbers indicate the order in which obstruction or constriction most often occurs. A myocardial infarction can involve only the endocardium or necrosis can penetrate all the way through the cardiac wall from the inner to the outer side. If necrosis is spread over a wide area, heart failure occurs within a short period of time. If sudden death does not occur, with time blood can begin to circulate again by developing connecting passages to nearby arterial branches. This is called collateral circulation.

Angina. When blood circulation is diminished because of narrowing of a coronary artery, a sudden increase in the work on the heart increases the oxygen demand and causes a serious state of oxygen deficiency to the heart muscle. Sharp pain is felt in the precordial region. Unlike myocardial infarction, the tissue does not die and recovery soon follows.

base of the aorta between the ventricles and the atria.

Extending from the aorta, the left coronary artery almost immediately divides into two branches, the circumflex branch and the anterior descending branch (anterior interventricular branch). The circumflex branch wraps around to the dorsal side approaching the right coronary artery, and the anterior descending branch extends toward the apex of the heart. These three major arteries widely supply the cardiac muscle and return to the right atrium via the venous system.

Features of Coronary Circulation. When the internal pressure of the heart is high because of cardiac contraction (systole), the coronary arteries become narrow, making it difficult for blood to circulate. Blood flows better when the ventricle relaxes (diastole) and the internal pressure is lowered. As a result, when the heartbeat is rapid (tachycardia), the contraction time becomes longer than the relaxation time, and the amount of blood supplied to the cardiac muscle decreases even though the work load is higher.

In coronary circulation, like the arteries of the four limbs, contraction and relaxation of the blood vessels is controlled by the autonomic nervous system (sympathetic and parasympathetic nervous system), but the reaction to command is weaker compared with the arteries of the four limbs. Thus when bleeding occurs in the arteries of the arms and legs or other internal organs, the muscles contract strongly and immediately reduce the flow of blood.

In contrast, the coronary arteries do not contract as strongly, so the flow of blood is relatively well maintained, enabling the heart to withstand the loss of blood. This is also characteristic of circulation in the brain, demonstrating the ingenious manner in which the heart and brain, which are vital to life, are protected.

Heart Rhythm and Cardiac Cycle

Electric impulses in the heart originate at the sinoatrial node of the right atrium, spread to the left and right atria, and make the atria contract. Next, the impulses travel to the atrioventricular node and are transmitted by the bundle of His (a special conduction system) and Purkinje's fibers to the ventricular muscle, resulting in contraction of the ventricle. There is no connection between the atria and ventricles: excitation in the atrium is transmitted by electric impulse through the bundle of His. The electrocardiographic waves below represent the electrical activity associated with depolarization of cardiac (atrial and ventricular) muscle and the progress of the impulse through the special conduction system. The cardiac cycle (the period between the start of one heartbeat and the beginning of the next) is also shown in the figure. In the electrocardiographic waves, the P wave is the impulse originating in the sinoatrial node and spreading through the atria. The QRS wave represents the activity associated with depolarization of the ventricles; it also reflects the time required for the impulse to spread through the bundle of His and its branches. The S-T segment represents the period between completion of ventricular depolarization and the start of repolarization. If the ventricular muscle is injured, as in acute myocardial infarction, the S-T segment may be elevated or depressed. The T wave represents the recovery phase following contraction. If the tissue is injured or ischemia is present, repolarization is abnormal, and the T wave may be inverted. The significance of the U wave remains unknown. In this figure, the period between the two P waves represents one cardiac cycle. If the heart beats 75 times per minute, one cardiac cycle requires approx 0.8 sec.

1. CONDUCTING SYSTEM OF THE HEART AND CARDIAC ACTIVITY

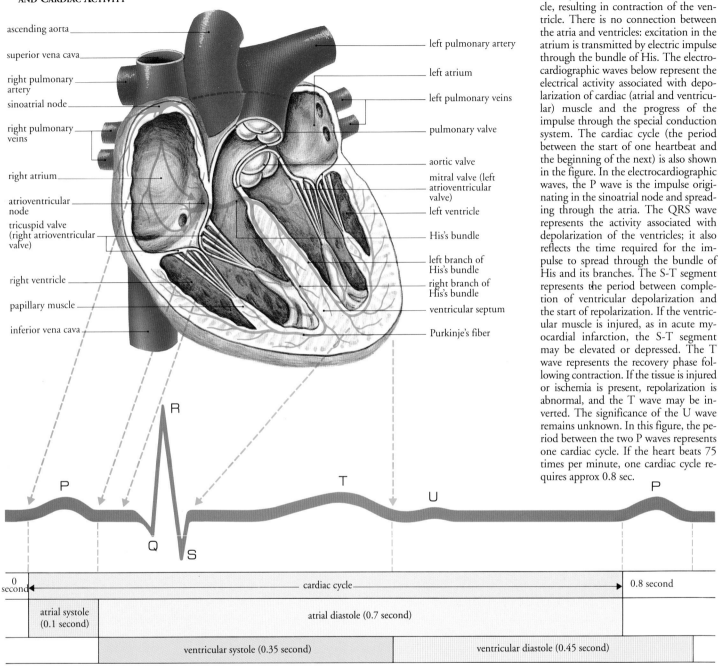

ascending aorta

superior vena cava

right pulmonary artery

sinoatrial node

right pulmonary veins

right atrium

atrioventricular node

tricuspid valve (right atrioventricular valve)

right ventricle

papillary muscle

inferior vena cava

left pulmonary artery

left atrium

left pulmonary veins

pulmonary valve

aortic valve

mitral valve (left atrioventricular valve)

left ventricle

His's bundle

left branch of His's bundle

right branch of His's bundle

ventricular septum

Purkinje's fiber

0 second	cardiac cycle		0.8 second
atrial systole (0.1 second)	atrial diastole (0.7 second)		
	ventricular systole (0.35 second)	ventricular diastole (0.45 second)	

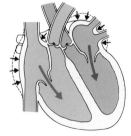

Blood filling the atria from the lungs and the rest of the body flows into the ventricles from the contraction of the atria.

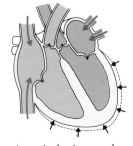

As atria begin to relax, the ventricles begin to contract. The tricuspid valve and the mitral valve close to prevent blood from flowing back into the atria. Pressure in the ventricles builds.

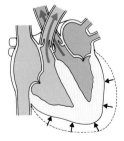

The ventricles contract. With build-up of internal pressure in the ventricles, the aortic and pulmonary valves are pushed open to allow blood to flow to the lungs and rest of the body.

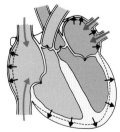

The ventricles begin to relax. The decrease in internal pressure causes the aortic and pulmonary valves to close, preventing blood from flowing back into the ventricles. Blood starts to flow into the atria.

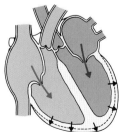

The atria fill up with blood from the lungs and the rest of the body. Rising internal atrial pressure pushes open the tricuspid and mitral valves, allowing blood to flow into the ventricles.

2. Ventricular Diastole and Systole

1. Ventricular Diastole

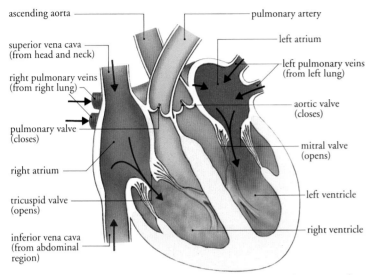

Internal pressure of the atria becomes higher than the internal pressure of the ventricles, pushing open the tricuspid and mitral valves and letting blood from the lungs and other parts of the body flow into the ventricles. Because the pressure of the aorta and pulmonary arteries is higher than the internal pressure of the ventricles, the aortic and pulmonary valves close, and the ventricular pressure reaches minimum. Blood pressure at ventricular relaxation (diastole) is the lowest blood pressure (diastolic pressure).

Intrinsic Rhythmicity and Conduction System of the Heart. Cardiac muscle cells have the ability to generate spontaneous and rhythmic electric impulses that are independent of any stimulus from nerves. Among the cardiac muscle cells, the sinoatrial node cells are the pacemaker because they have the fastest rhythm. The cardiac muscle cells involved in the conduction system differ in function from ordinary cardiac muscle. The function of ordinary cardiac muscle is contraction and relaxation and, like all other muscle, it can also conduct impulses. Conduction alone is the special function of the modified cardiac muscle cells that comprise the conduction system. Four structures—the sinoatrial node, atrioventricular node, atrioventricular bundle, and Purkinje fibers—comprise the conduction system of the heart. The electric signals occurring in the sinoatrial node are transmitted radially throughout the atria and collect in the sinoatrial node. From there the signals travel to the bundle of His, the left and right branches of the bundle of His, the Purkinje fibers, and the ventricular muscle (from inner wall to outer wall). In the embryo, the heart begins to beat long before any nerves have grown out to it. The property of this autonomic rhythmic contractibility is so highly developed in cardiac muscle that if a heart is maintained under proper conditions it will continue to beat after removal from the body. It must be kept oxygenated in a balanced solution of sodium, potassium, and calcium chloride and maintained at a temperature of 37°C.

Electrocardiogram. As with all muscles, cardiac muscle generates action potential. Every beat of the heart is accompanied by an electrical change. Electrolytes in the body fluids and tissues act as conductors to the skin surface; metal leads applied to the skin thus can conduct the current to an instrument that makes a graphic tracing of the activity. The tracing during each cardiac cycle is characterized by five waves, which are arbitrarily designated as P, Q, R, S, and T. Occasionally, the U wave appears. This tracing is the electrocardiogram, and it provides information regarding the electrical activity of the heart. Although it is a valuable

2. Ventricular Systole

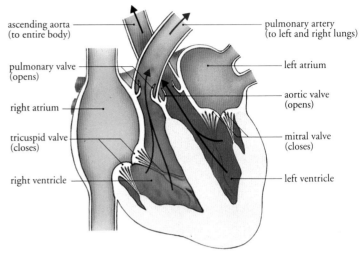

When internal pressure in the ventricles rises, the tricuspid and mitral valves close, preventing incoming blood from flowing back into the atria. When the internal ventricular pressure becomes higher than the pressure in the aorta and pulmonary arteries, the aortic and pulmonary valves are pushed open, the ventricles contract further and, with maximum pressure, send blood out to the lungs and other parts of the body. The blood pressure at ventricular contraction (systole) is the highest blood pressure (systolic pressure).

diagnostic tool, it does not reflect the pumping ability of the heart.

Electrocardiographic Variation. If the demand for blood by the cardiac muscles exceeds the supply or circulation is obstructed (infarction), a change occurs in the conducting system or in the process of cardiac muscle contraction and relaxation, resulting in electrocardiographic variation. Electrocardiographic variations can also occur as a result of disorders in generation of excitation in cardiac muscles (arrhythmia, flutter, fibrillation, ectopic rhythm), hypertrophy, and changes in electrolyte level in blood, making electrocardiograms useful for the diagnosis of these disorders.

Cardiac Cycle. The left and right atria and ventricles contract and relax in the same cardiac cycle. A slight time lapse occurs between the contractions of the atria and ventricles. These contractions and relaxations are broadly divided into systole and diastole. The cycle of a single systole and diastole (contraction and relaxation) is known as the cardiac cycle. The atrioventricular valve located between the left and right atria and ventricles closes just before the beginning of a ventricular contraction, and the arterial valves (pulmonary valve, aortic valve) close toward the end of the ventricular contraction. The atrioventricular valve opens during ventricular diastole, and the pulmonary valve opens during ventricular systole.

Malformation of the Heart. The heart forms in the embryonic stage (the period when the fetus is developing in the uterus) from a single cylindrical mass of tissue that twists and divides as it forms. It is a complex process and malformations sometimes occur. For example, various valve malformations can occur, the septum between the left and right atria and ventricles can close in completely (atrial septal defect, ventricular septal defect), or the arteries that should close at the end of development remain open (patent ductus arteriosus). These are cases of congenital cardiopathy.

Major Disorders: angina, myocardial infarction, pericarditis, valvular diseases, atrioventricular block, congenital heart disorder (atrial septal defect, ventricular septal defect, patent ductus arteriosus), Fallot's tetralogy.

The Breast

1. Breast of Pregnant Woman (cutaway section)

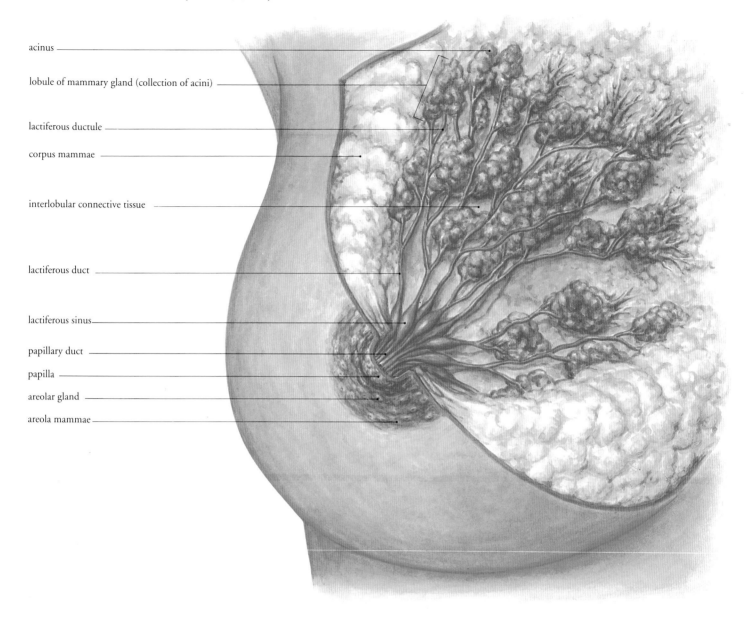

acinus

lobule of mammary gland (collection of acini)

lactiferous ductule

corpus mammae

interlobular connective tissue

lactiferous duct

lactiferous sinus

papillary duct

papilla

areolar gland

areola mammae

The breasts function as part of the reproductive system, but structurally they are appendages of the skin. In males and prepubescent females, the breasts take the form of small nipples resembling buds. In postpubescent females, the breasts are larger, and after the birth of a baby, breasts secrete milk, playing a vital role in the growth and development of the infant.

Location. Located at the front of the thoracic region, the breasts develop between the second and sixth ribs, from the edge of the thoracic bone to the anterior border line of the axilla. In some mammals numerous breasts develop along the mammary ridge connecting the axilla and the groin, but in most humans only a single pair (the fourth pair) develops.

Size and Shape. Size and shape of breasts varies by sex, age, and whether or not one is pregnant or nursing. In addition, individual differences are great. In females, the mammary glands develop at puberty when secretion of estrogen increases. The subcutaneous adipose tissue surrounding the mammary glands increases and the breasts grow semicircular in shape.

Structure. Mammary cells that secrete milk collect to form alveoli, at the base of which are myoepithelial cells. Groups of alveoli form lobules from which milk is secreted. The milk is stored in lactiferous sinuses and excreted through lactiferous ducts.

The nipple is found toward the center of each breast, surrounded by a pigmented area called an areola. When pregnancy occurs, the pigment melanin is deposited, and the pink color diminishes as the areola becomes darker. There are about 20 openings to lactiferous ducts located at the nipple, and areolar glands and a small number of sweat glands are also located on the areola.

Excretion of Milk. During pregnancy, the lobules of the mammary gland develop in response to changing levels of estrogen and other hormones. After delivery, the hormone prolactin begins to stimulate the excretion of milk. When the baby sucks on the nipple, the action stimulates contraction of the muscle tissue around the mammary gland and milk is expressed.

Major Disorders: mastitis, mastopathy, fibroadenoma, breast cancer, abnormal lactation.

2. LOCATION OF MAMMARY RIDGE AND ACCESSORY MAMMAE

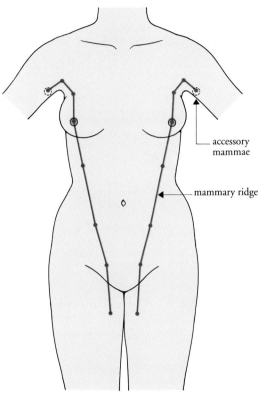

accessory mammae

mammary ridge

In some mammals, numerous breasts develop on two mammary ridges, which run vertically along the anterior of the body. In humans, only the fourth pair from the top develop, the others having degenerated. Cases in which additional small breasts developed along the ridge have been recognized, however. These additional breasts are known as accessory breasts, or polymastia.

3. HOW MILK IS SECRETED

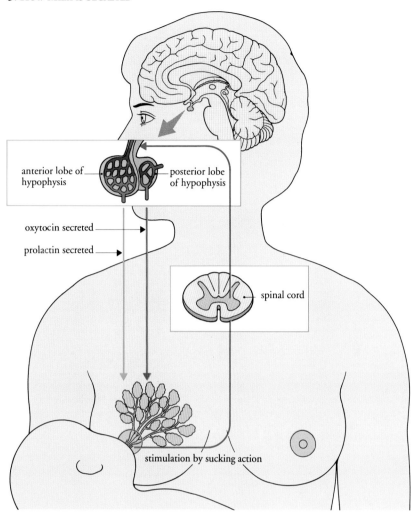

anterior lobe of hypophysis

posterior lobe of hypophysis

oxytocin secreted

prolactin secreted

spinal cord

stimulation by sucking action

Lactation involves the two processes of production and expression of milk. The sucking action of the infant on the mother's nipple causes the sensory nerves of the papillae to stimulate via the spinal cord, the pituitary gland. As a result of this stimulation, prolactin is excreted from the anterior lobe and oxytocin from the posterior lobe. Prolactin promotes the production of milk, and oxytocin aids in its excretion by making the muscle tissue around the mammary gland contract to push the milk through the lactiferous ducts to the papillae and from there into the baby's mouth.

4. PATHOLOGY OF MASTITIS

1. Parenchymatous Mastitis

2. Interstitial Mastitis

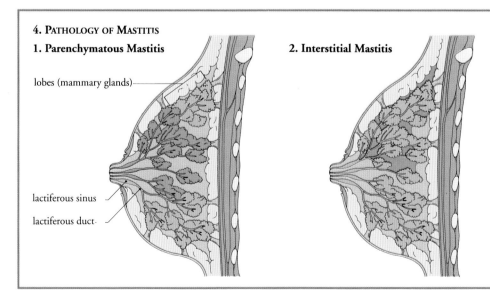

lobes (mammary glands)

lactiferous sinus

lactiferous duct

Mastitis is an inflammation of the mammary gland caused by infection. It is characterized by redness, swelling, and pain of the breasts or surrounding skin. Sometimes mastitis is accompanied by symptoms such as high fever and chills. Mastitis almost always occurs in the period immediately following childbirth (the puerperal period). Abscesses may develop in severe cases. Mastitis is classified based on where the inflammation occurs. In parenchymatous mastitis, the inflammation occurs first in the lactiferous ducts and spreads to the mammary glands. In interstitial mastitis, the inflammation occurs in the spaces between the lobes of the mammary glands. The parts shown in gray indicate where inflammation can occur.

3 | The Abdominal Region

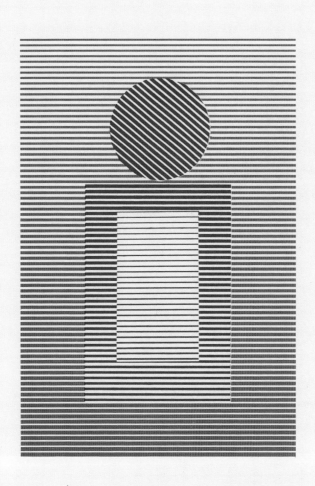

The Abdomen

The abdomen houses the organs of the digestive system (digestion and absorption), the urinary system (filtering and discharging wastes from the body), and the reproductive organs (procreation).

Abdomen Contents. The diaphragm separates the thorax from the abdomen. Below and to the right of the diaphragm (which is shaped like a large pan turned upside down) is the largest organ in the body, the liver; the stomach is below and to the left of the diaphragm and farther to the left is the spleen. The small intestine, large intestine, and urinary bladder are located below the liver and stomach, and the kidneys are situated in the rear.

A cage-like structure made up of the ribs, sternum, and backbone protects the organs of the thorax from external injury. The abdominal organs of four-footed mammals are protected against injury from the rear by the pelvic wall and backbone. The four limbs also provide protection by fencing in the abdomen.

Standing upright on two feet, humans have undergone marvelous evolutionary development with regard to intelligence, but this occurred at the expense of exposing the abdomen, leaving it unprotected against enemy attack and other dangers.

ABDOMINAL CAVITY AND PERITONEUM. The abdominal organs are classified according to those found within the abdominal cavity and completely enclosed by the peritoneum (stomach, jejunum, ileum, gallbladder, transverse colon, sigmoid colon, ovaries, fallopian tubes), those partially enclosed by the peritoneum (liver, ascending colon, descending colon, rectum, uterus, bladder), and those that lie farther to the rear in the posterior peritoneal cavity (kidneys, adrenal glands, pancreas).

The upper parts of the uterus, urinary bladder, and rectum are covered by the peritoneum and located in the pelvic region. When pregnancy occurs, the uterus becomes enlarged and protrudes into the abdominal cavity. When a lot of urine fills the bladder, it becomes enlarged along the anterior abdominal wall. The ureters, anal canal, rectum, spermiduct, and seminal vesicle in males, and the vagina in females, is located below the abdomen in the lower part of the pelvic region called the true pelvis.

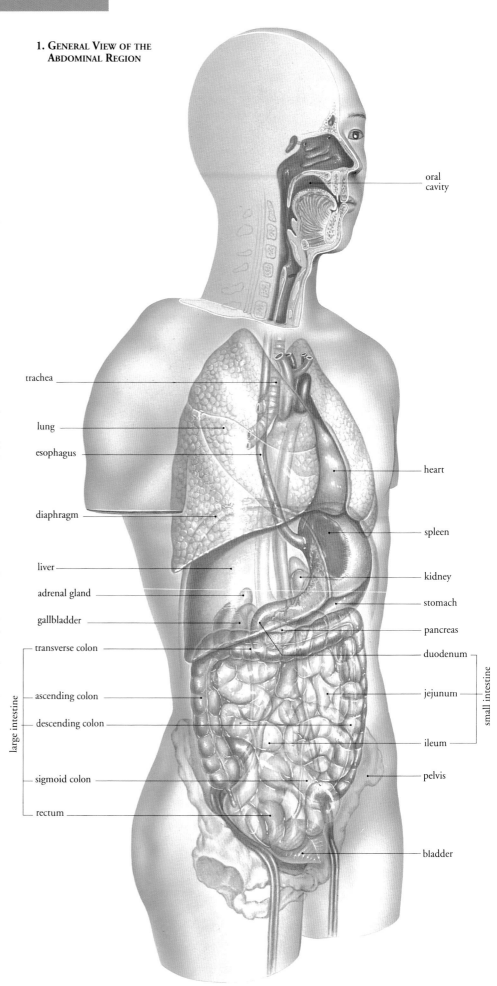

1. GENERAL VIEW OF THE ABDOMINAL REGION

oral cavity

trachea

lung

esophagus

heart

diaphragm

spleen

liver

kidney

adrenal gland

stomach

gallbladder

pancreas

transverse colon

duodenum

ascending colon

jejunum

descending colon

ileum

sigmoid colon

pelvis

rectum

bladder

large intestine

small intestine

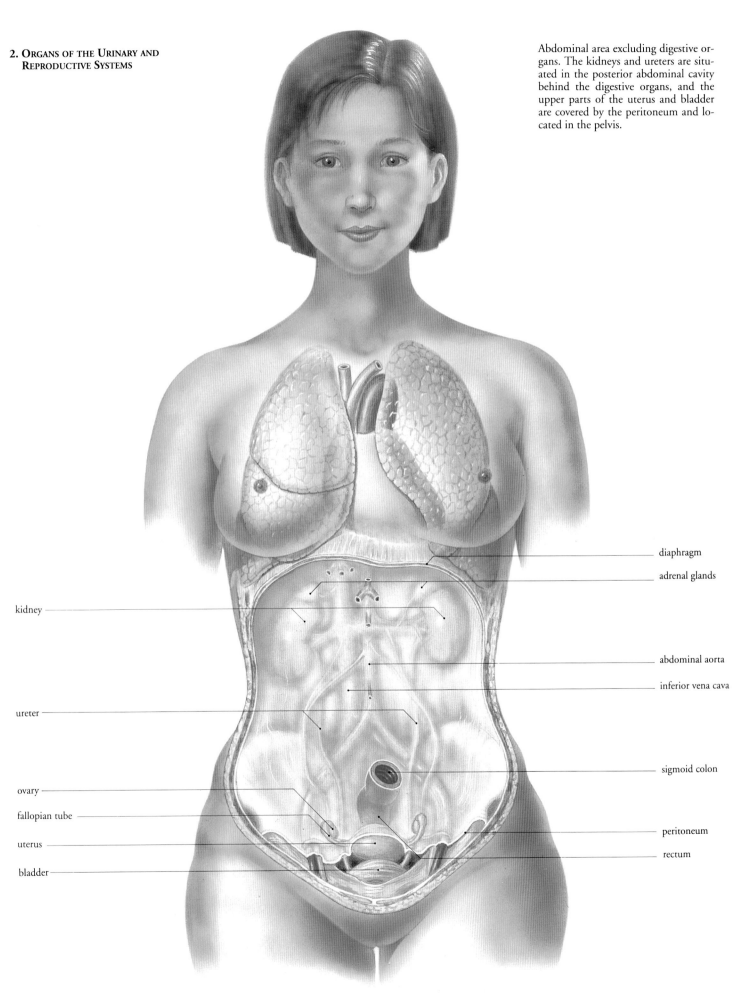

2. ORGANS OF THE URINARY AND REPRODUCTIVE SYSTEMS

Abdominal area excluding digestive organs. The kidneys and ureters are situated in the posterior abdominal cavity behind the digestive organs, and the upper parts of the uterus and bladder are covered by the peritoneum and located in the pelvis.

kidney

ureter

ovary

fallopian tube

uterus

bladder

diaphragm

adrenal glands

abdominal aorta

inferior vena cava

sigmoid colon

peritoneum

rectum

The Esophagus

3. ORGANS OF THE DIGESTIVE SYSTEM

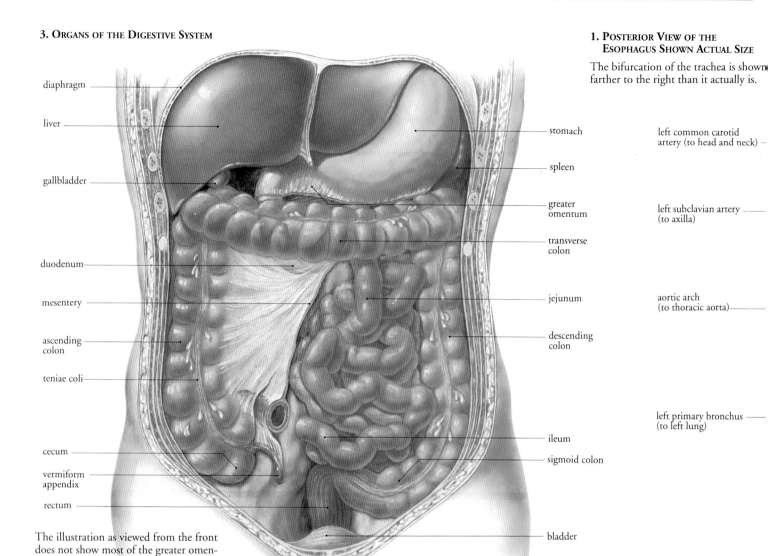

diaphragm

liver

gallbladder

duodenum

mesentery

ascending colon

teniae coli

cecum

vermiform appendix

rectum

stomach

spleen

greater omentum

transverse colon

jejunum

descending colon

ileum

sigmoid colon

bladder

The illustration as viewed from the front does not show most of the greater omentum, the right half of the mesentery, or part of the small intestine (ileum).

1. POSTERIOR VIEW OF THE ESOPHAGUS SHOWN ACTUAL SIZE

The bifurcation of the trachea is shown farther to the right than it actually is.

left common carotid artery (to head and neck)

left subclavian artery (to axilla)

aortic arch (to thoracic aorta)

left primary bronchus (to left lung)

Arrangement of the Alimentary Canal.

The lower part of the stomach adjacent to the lower right portion of the diaphragm is connected to the pylorus, the opening that leads from the stomach to a part of the small intestine called the duodenum. The larger part of the duodenum, which is connected to the stomach, is attached to the posterior peritoneal wall. The jejunum and ileum (additional sections of the small intestine) border the mesentery. The base of the mesentery attaches the small intestine to the posterior abdominal wall, so movement is somewhat limited. The jejunum is located mainly in the upper left part of the abdomen and the ileum is found in the lower right section.

The ileum is attached to the ascending colon of the large intestine at nearly a right angle. The large intestine (ascending, transverse, and descending colon) winds in an "M" formation around the upper midsection of the abdomen to become the sigmoid colon, which ends with the rectum and anus.

The esophagus transports food and liquid from the mouth to the stomach.

Location. From the pharynx the esophagus passes near the larynx between the trachea and the spinal column and through the mediastinum of the chest wall. Passing behind the heart and through the diaphragm, it enters the abdomen and connects with the stomach.

Size and Shape. It is a long passage 25 cm in length and 2 cm in diameter. When food is not traveling through, the passage is nearly closed because of the crossfolds of the mucous membrane.

Structure. The esophagus comprises two layers of muscle, circular muscles on the inside and longitudinal muscles on the outside. The internal surface of muscle is lined with mucous membrane and the external surface is covered by a flexible tectorial membrane. The lower two-thirds of the muscle of the esophagus is smooth muscle and the upper one-third is made up of striated muscle, or skeletal muscle.

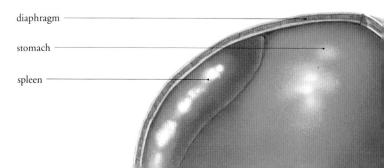

diaphragm

stomach

spleen

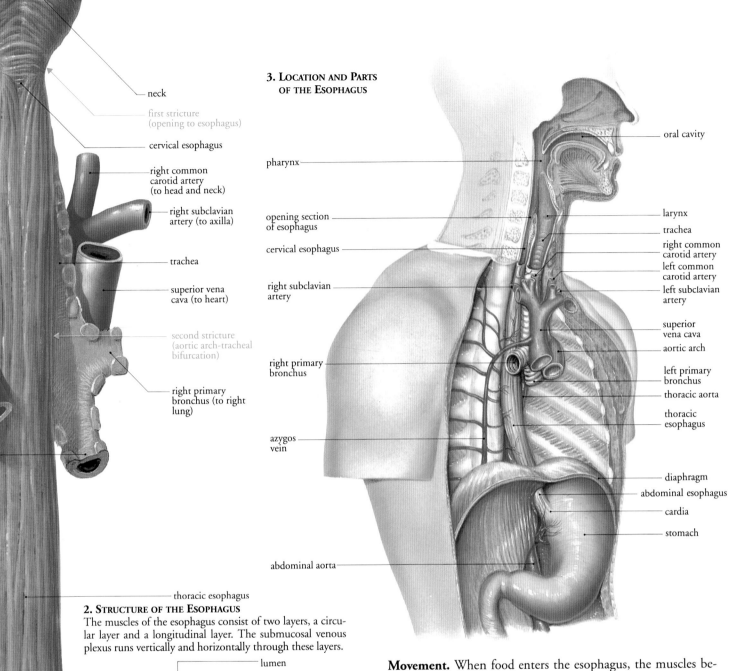

neck

first stricture
(opening to esophagus)

cervical esophagus

right common
carotid artery
(to head and neck)

right subclavian
artery (to axilla)

trachea

superior vena
cava (to heart)

second stricture
(aortic arch-tracheal
bifurcation)

right primary
bronchus (to right
lung)

3. LOCATION AND PARTS OF THE ESOPHAGUS

pharynx

opening section
of esophagus

cervical esophagus

right subclavian
artery

right primary
bronchus

azygos
vein

abdominal aorta

oral cavity

larynx

trachea

right common
carotid artery

left common
carotid artery

left subclavian
artery

superior
vena cava

aortic arch

left primary
bronchus

thoracic aorta

thoracic
esophagus

diaphragm

abdominal esophagus

cardia

stomach

thoracic esophagus

2. STRUCTURE OF THE ESOPHAGUS

The muscles of the esophagus consist of two layers, a circular layer and a longitudinal layer. The submucosal venous plexus runs vertically and horizontally through these layers.

lumen

mucosal tunic
of esophagus

muscular layer
of mucosa

submucosal
venous plexus

submucosa

circular
muscle

longitudinal
muscle

muscular tunic of esophagus

third stricture (esophageal hiatus)

thoracic artery (to abdominal artery)

Movement. When food enters the esophagus, the muscles begin their peristaltic action, and the resulting wavelike motion pushes the food downward toward the stomach. The striated muscles in the upper part of the esophagus function on a voluntary basis, but when the food reaches the part of the esophagus covered with only smooth muscle, an involuntary (swallowing) reflex occurs in response to stimulation of the esophageal wall, resulting in continuation of peristalsis. At the boundary between the esophagus (cardia) and the stomach, smooth muscles are well developed and function as a sphincter to prevent backflow of food from the stomach. The time required for food to pass through the esophagus is 1–6 sec for liquids and 30–60 sec for solid foods mixed well with saliva.

Major Disorders: Esophagitis, cancer of the esophagus, esophageal varix, esophageal stenosis.

The Stomach and Duodenum

- **Stomach:** Size (with average content): greater curvature approx 49 cm; lesser curvature approx 13 cm, volume (when full): approx 1200–1600 ml
- **Duodenum:** Length: approx 30 cm

1. The Stomach Shown Actual Size

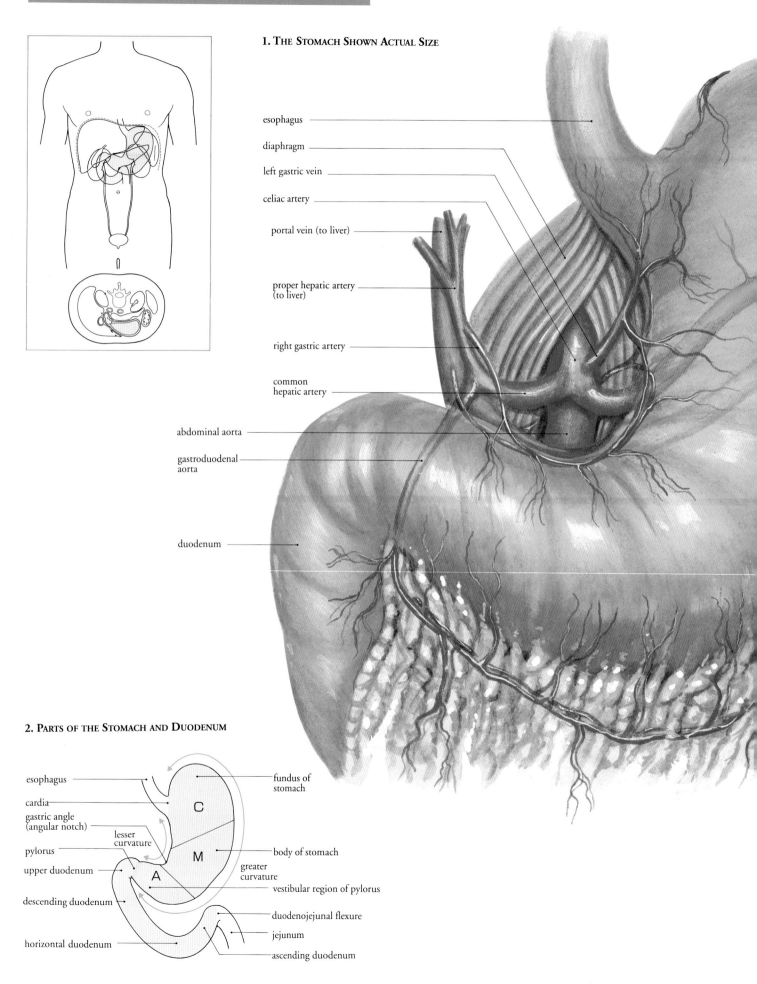

esophagus

diaphragm

left gastric vein

celiac artery

portal vein (to liver)

proper hepatic artery (to liver)

right gastric artery

common hepatic artery

abdominal aorta

gastroduodenal aorta

duodenum

2. Parts of the Stomach and Duodenum

esophagus

cardia

gastric angle (angular notch)

lesser curvature

pylorus

upper duodenum

descending duodenum

horizontal duodenum

fundus of stomach

body of stomach

greater curvature

vestibular region of pylorus

duodenojejunal flexure

jejunum

ascending duodenum

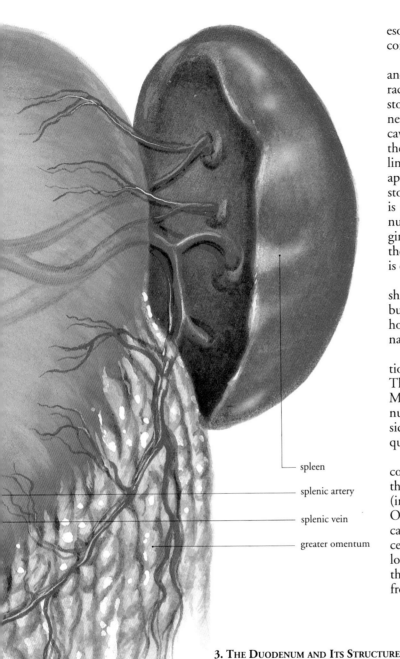

The stomach temporarily stores food entering through the esophagus so that the first stage of digestion can begin. Digestion continues in the duodenum.

Location. The stomach occupies most of the area to the left and below the diaphragm, which is the border between the thoracic and abdominal regions. The liver is located to the right of the stomach. Together, these two organs take up most of the space beneath the diaphragm. Most of the remaining area of the abdominal cavity is occupied by the small and large intestines. The fundus of the stomach is in contact with the heart through the several millimeters of the diaphragm. The esophagus passes through the diaphragm and joins the stomach. The spleen lies to the right of the stomach, and the pancreas lies below and to the rear; the pancreas is positioned as if its front section were being held by the duodenum. The duodenum is the first part of the small intestine. It begins at the outlet of the stomach (pylorus) and is held in place at the rear of the abdominal wall by the peritoneum. The duodenum is curved in a horseshoe shape and connects to the jejunum.

Size and Shape. The stomach has been described as having the shape of an upside down bull horn. Its size varies with content, but when it is full its volume is approx 1200–1600 ml. The horseshoe shaped duodenum is about 30 cm in length. It is so named because it is about the length of twelve finger breadths.

The Parts of the Stomach. To clearly and easily indicate location, the stomach is divided into sections (as shown in Figure 2). The fundus is marked C, the body of the stomach is designated M, and the pyloric is marked part A. Another method is to use numbers to indicate the site. The part of the duodenum just outside the pylorus is called the upper duodenum, and the subsequent parts are labeled in the figure.

Structure of the Duodenum. The duodenum is completely covered by the peritoneum. Its layers, from the inside out, include the mucous membrane, submucosa glands, two layers of muscle (inner circular layer and outer longitudinal layer), and the serosa. On the surface of the mucous membrane are circular folds, or plical. Each plica is covered with thin projections called villi and cells that secrete various hormones. The major duodenal papilla is located near the center of the descending duodenum. This marks the location of the ampulla of Vater, the common bile duct leading from the liver (and sometimes the pancreas) to the duodenum.

spleen

splenic artery

splenic vein

greater omentum

3. THE DUODENUM AND ITS STRUCTURE

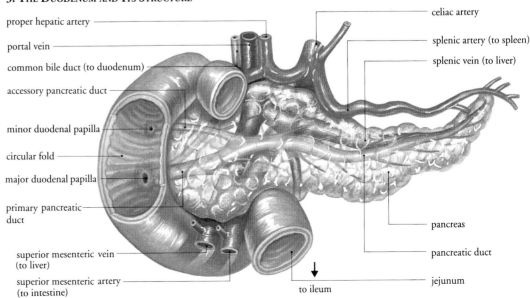

proper hepatic artery

portal vein

common bile duct (to duodenum)

accessory pancreatic duct

minor duodenal papilla

circular fold

major duodenal papilla

primary pancreatic duct

superior mesenteric vein (to liver)

superior mesenteric artery (to intestine)

celiac artery

splenic artery (to spleen)

splenic vein (to liver)

pancreas

pancreatic duct

jejunum

to ileum

The pancreas is located to the rear of the stomach, and the front is covered by the duodenum, which is in the shape of the letter "C." The common bile duct and primary pancreatic duct, which are passages for digestive fluids, join and open into the duodenum.

4. MUSCLES OF THE STOMACH

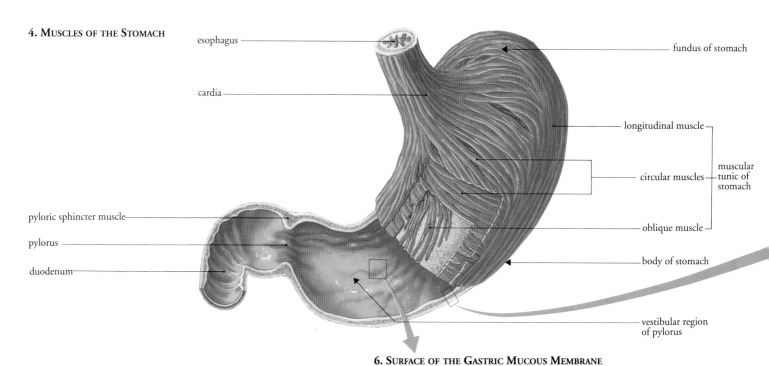

esophagus

cardia

fundus of stomach

longitudinal muscle

circular muscles — muscular tunic of stomach

oblique muscle

pyloric sphincter muscle

pylorus

duodenum

body of stomach

vestibular region of pylorus

5. INSIDE THE STOMACH

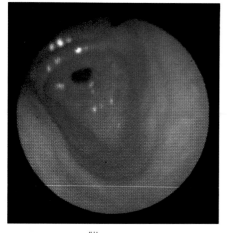

This is the interior of a normal stomach viewed through an endoscope. The black spot seen at upper left is the pylorus. The diagram below the photograph shows the location of the endoscope and the area viewed.

6. SURFACE OF THE GASTRIC MUCOUS MEMBRANE VIEWED THROUGH A SCANNING ELECTRON MICROSCOPE

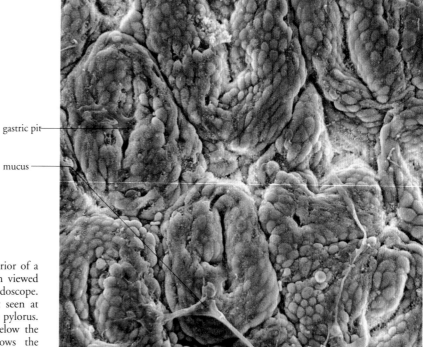

gastric pit

mucus

0.02mm

7. EXPANSION AND MOVEMENT OF THE STOMACH

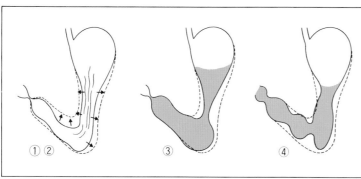

① ② ③ ④

① When the stomach is empty, the rugae, or folds, of the inner surface of the stomach narrow lengthwise much like a bellows.

② As the amount of food in the stomach increases, these folds stretch and expand.

③ As food falls into the body of the stomach and accumulates, waves of contractions churn the food and begin to transport it.

④ The contents of the stomach are then moved into the duodenum by contractions of the pylorus.

8. Structure of the Stomach Wall

gastric pit

gastric gland

capillary

muco-epidermis

proper mucous membrane

mucous membrane

muscular layer of mucosa

submucosa

muscular tunic of stomach

serosa

Structure of the Stomach. The stomach is basically a pouch made up of three layers of smooth muscle. The innermost layer is the oblique layer, in which muscle fibers run in a diagonal direction, the middle layer is the circular layer, which consists of fibers encircling the stomach, and the outermost layer is made up of the longitudinal layer in which muscle fibers run lengthwise along the stomach. The circular layer is particularly well developed at the pylorus, becoming the pyloric sphincter muscle. The muscular tunic of the stomach is lined by a mucous membrane (mucoepidermis, proper mucous membrane, muscular layer of mucosa) and submucosa, and the outside of the tunic is covered by the serosa and the peritoneum. Almost all stomach ulcers and malignant tumors start in the mucous membrane and grow toward the serosa.

Movement. The stomach mixes and transports its contents by contracting and relaxing in regular segmental, pendular, and peristaltic movements. One contraction lasts from 2–20 sec, and a maximum of 3–5 contractions occurs each min. In addition to the peristaltic movement that moves food toward the pylorus, peristaltic movement occurs in the pyloric part of the stomach in the opposite direction to mix food and gastric juices. Normally food from one meal takes about 4 hr to go from the stomach to the duodenum, but it can take longer if the meal includes fatty food. The duodenum has peristaltic movement toward the jejunum.

Function. The stomach temporarily stores the food that comes through the esophagus and in coordination with the progress in digestion being made in the small intestine (especially in the duodenum) sends it on to the duodenum. The stomach also acts as an agitator to thoroughly mix the food and gastric juices.

The duodenum adds pancreatic juice and bile to the food that has been prepared for digestion by the stomach so it can be easily absorbed in the small and large intestines.

Excretory Juices. Gastric juice is excreted from the mucous membrane of the stomach. Gastric juice is made up of hydrochloric acid, the digestive enzyme pepsin, and mucus. The hydrochloric acid is strongly acidic, with pH of 1.0–2.5. Mucus prevents the muscles of the stomach from being dissolved by the action of the gastric juice as it digests protein in the stomach. Approximately 1500–2500 ml of gastric juice is excreted per day. Alkaline intestinal juice, which includes various kinds of digestive enzymes and different alimentary hormones, is excreted from the mucous membrane of the duodenum.

Major Disorders: gastritis, stomach ulcer, gastric polyps, stomach cancer, gastroptosis, gastric atony, duodenal ulcer, duodenal diverticulum, cancer of the major duodenal papilla.

The Small Intestine, Large Intestine and Anus

•**Small Intestine:** Length: approx 6.35–7 m (in the living body)
•**Large Intestine:** Length: approx 1.5 m
•**Rectum:** Length: approx 15 cm
•**Vermiform Appendix:** Length: approx 6–9 cm

1. Section of the Abdominal Region

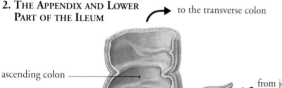

diaphragm
liver
lesser omentum
pancreas
stomach
mesentery of transverse colon
transverse colon
peritoneum
greater omentum
small intestine
bladder
prostate
anus

celiac artery
superior mesentery artery
abdominal aorta
duodenum
inferior mesentery artery
mesentery
posterior peritoneum
rectum

The organs of the digestive system are enveloped by the peritoneum, and the small and large intestines are connected to the mesentery, which is attached to the rear of the peritoneal wall.

2. The Appendix and Lower Part of the Ileum

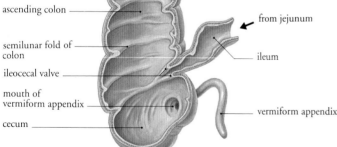

to the transverse colon

ascending colon
semilunar fold of colon
ileocecal valve
mouth of vermiform appendix
cecum

from jejunum
ileum
vermiform appendix

3. The Mesentery and Distribution of the Arteries and Veins

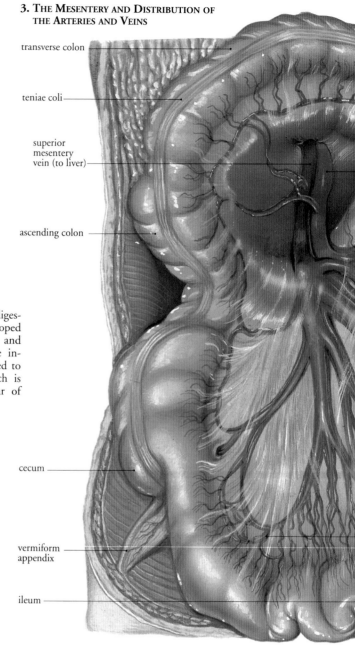

transverse colon
teniae coli
superior mesentery vein (to liver)
ascending colon
cecum
vermiform appendix
ileum

SMALL INTESTINE

The small intestine, which plays a major role in the digestive system, is the long canal that digests and absorbs chyme—food that has been churned with gastric juice and turned into a thick soupy fluid in the stomach.

Location. The small intestine is made up of three parts: the duodenum, which extends from the stomach opening (pylorus), the jejunum, and the ileum. The duodenum is fixed to the posterior abdominal wall, but the remaining parts of the small intestine and the large intestine occupy most of the abdominal cavity.

Size. The small intestine is a soft canal about 7 m in length, as measured in the body, with a diameter about the size of a half-dollar coin. The jejunum makes up about two-fifths of the small intestine, and the ileum makes up the remaining three-fifths. The ileum is somewhat wider than the jejunum and has a thicker wall that is pinkish in color.

Structure. The small intestine has an inner lining of mucous membrane surrounded by a muscular tunic (an inner layer of circular muscles and outer layer of longitudinal muscles). The peritoneum covers this outer muscular layer. Circular folds called plicae are found in the mucous membrane (these are especially numerous in the jejunum), and villi grow on the surface. In addition, on each villi grows an average of 600 microvilli, making the internal surface area extremely large.

MESENTERY. The mesentery is the membrane that attaches the intestines to the posterior wall of the abdominal cavity. It is a very thin membrane formed by peritoneum that comes together from the two sides of the abdomen. Blood vessels can be seen running through the mesentery. The part that is fixed to the posterior abdominal wall is narrow in width, about 15 cm, but it spreads out and widens into a fan shape of about 3 cm. The jejunum and ileum are attached to this fan-shaped part of the mesentery, forming a kind of apron, and the blood vessels, lymphatic vessels, and nerves run through the mesentery to reach the small intestine.

LARGE INTESTINE

Location. The large intestine is broadly divided into the cecum, colon, and rectum. The colon is made up of the ascending, transverse, descending, and sigmoid colon. The ascending colon goes upward from the cecum to the right inferior abdominal re-

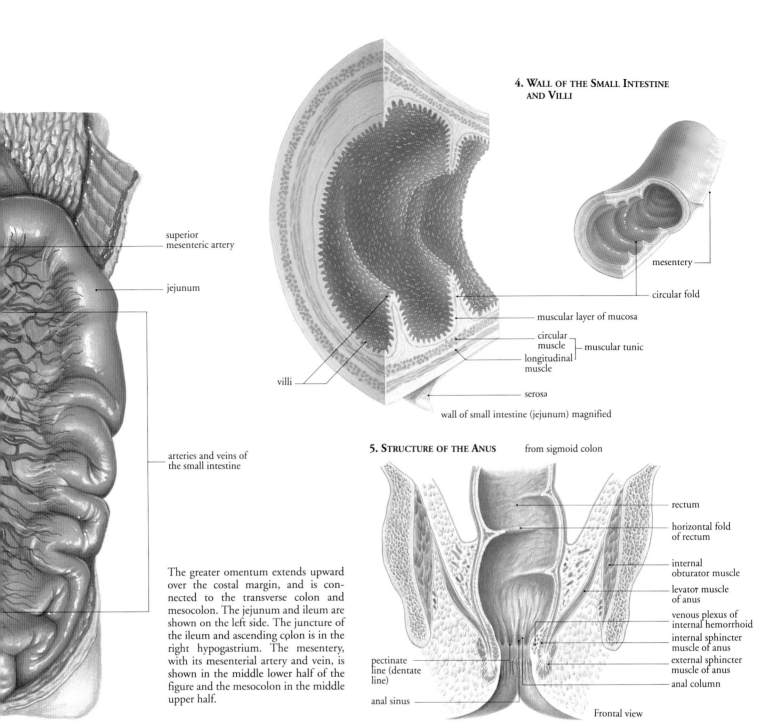

superior mesenteric artery

jejunum

arteries and veins of the small intestine

villi

mesentery

circular fold

muscular layer of mucosa

circular muscle — muscular tunic
longitudinal muscle

serosa

wall of small intestine (jejunum) magnified

5. STRUCTURE OF THE ANUS from sigmoid colon

rectum

horizontal fold of rectum

internal obturator muscle

levator muscle of anus

venous plexus of internal hemorrhoid

internal sphincter muscle of anus

external sphincter muscle of anus

anal column

pectinate line (dentate line)

anal sinus

Frontal view

The greater omentum extends upward over the costal margin, and is connected to the transverse colon and mesocolon. The jejunum and ileum are shown on the left side. The juncture of the ileum and ascending colon is in the right hypogastrium. The mesentery, with its mesenterial artery and vein, is shown in the middle lower half of the figure and the mesocolon in the middle upper half.

gion. The colon turns left and becomes the descending colon, which comes down the left side of the abdominal region. The sigmoid colon ends at the rectum, where it joins the anus. The ascending and descending colons are fixed to the posterior abdominal wall, but the transverse colon, which hangs from the long mesocolon, is able to move somewhat.

Size, Shape, and Structure. The large intestine is about 1.5 m in length, and its width is two to three times that of the small intestine. In contrast to the small intestine, its outward appearance is not smooth. Three bands of longitudinal muscles, each 8 mm in width, are attached at equal intervals, making the colon take on a kind of loose bellows formation.

The end of the ileum of the small intestine and the ascending colon are joined in a T formation. At this juncture the ileum protrudes somewhat to form the ileocecal valve, which prevents the contents of the large intestine from flowing back into the small intestine. The tail end of this juncture is the appendix, at the end of which there hangs the vermiform appendix, which resembles a rather fat worm.

Functions of the Small and Large Intestines. Most of the functions related to digestion and absorption are done in the small intestine. The large intestine absorbs about one-fourth of the fluid from the contents that have been transported from the ileum. The large intestine also absorbs sodium and various salts, and discharges potassium.

RECTUM AND ANUS

The rectum, at the end of the large intestine, is approx 15 cm long. It has three horizontal folds that function as valves. Stool is stored in the sigmoid colon, moves into the rectum as a result of general muscle contraction that occurs several times a day, and is discharged in a bowel movement.

The internal anal sphincter muscle located at the inner side of the anus is smooth muscle and subject to involuntary movement, but the external anal sphincter muscle, aided by striated muscles, moves on a voluntary basis. The two sphincter muscles work together to open and close the anus.

Major Disorders: appendicitis, intestinal obstruction, irritable bowel syndrome, polyps, colon and rectal cancer, hemorrhoids, anal fistula, etc.

Digestion and Absorption—The Wall of the Digestive Tract

Throughout the inner wall of the digestive tract, which extends from the esophagus through the stomach and the small and large intestines, glands secrete mucus. This aids the "belt conveyor" mechanism of peristalsis in smoothly transporting food that has been ingested. In addition there are other glands that secrete various digestive juices in the stomach and small intestine.

The primary roles of the stomach are the digestion of proteins and the prevention of putrefaction by the strong hydrochloric acid in gastric juice. Water and alcohol are the only substances absorbed by the stomach. In the small intestine, pancreatic juice (produced in the pancreas) and bile (produced in the liver) are secreted in the duodenum along with digestive juices produced in the small intestine itself. In addition to peristaltic motion, agitation of food in the form of articulate pendular motion also occurs. Moreover, the mixing of these digestive juices with food is enhanced by the folds (plicae) of the small intestine and on villi, whose surfaces have been further expanded by the microvilli. The digestion that occurs in the large intestine is minimal, limited mainly to absorption of water and electrolytes.

1. GENERAL VIEW OF DIGESTIVE TRACT

- oral cavity
- pharynx
- esophagus
  Food passes through in approximately 30–60 seconds and liquids in 1–6 seconds.
- stomach
  approx 4 hours
- duodenum
- small intestine (jejunum, ileum)
  approx 7–9 hours
- large intestine (colon)
  approx 25–30 hours
- rectum
  approx 30–120 hours

2. MUCOUS MEMBRANE OF THE DIGESTIVE TRACT

1. Esophagus, Stomach, Duodenum

- mucous membrane of esophagus
- cardia
- fold of gastric mucous membrane
- pylorus
- fold of mucous membrane of duodenum

3. STRUCTURE OF THE WALL OF THE DIGESTIVE TRACT

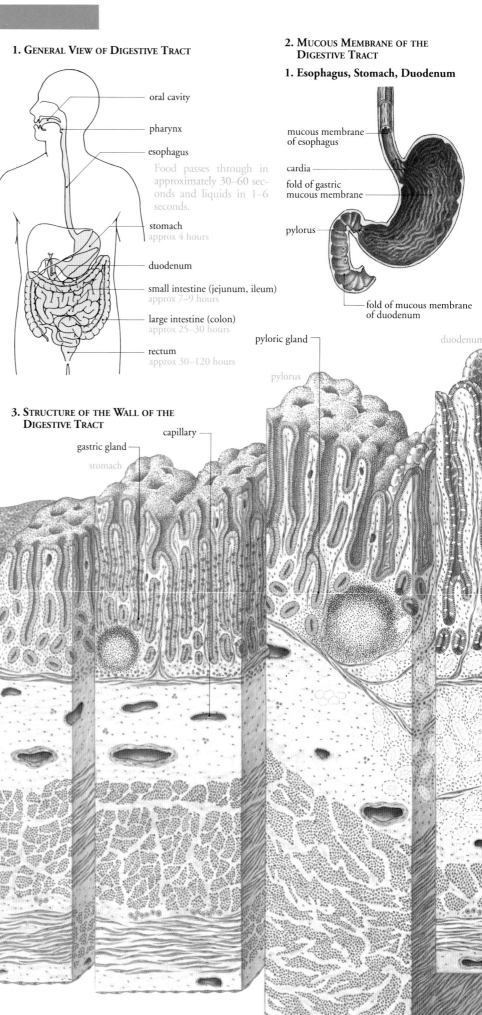

esophageal gland
excretory duct
esophagus
cardia
stomach
gastric gland
capillary
pyloric gland
pylorus
duodenum

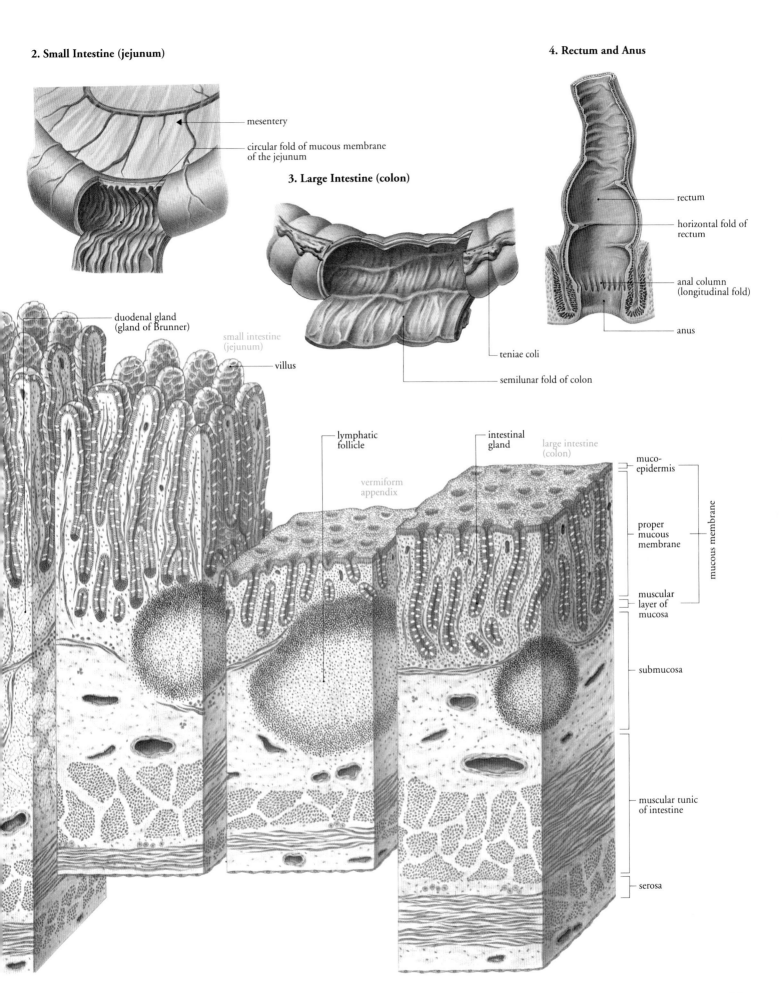

2. Small Intestine (jejunum)

mesentery

circular fold of mucous membrane
of the jejunum

3. Large Intestine (colon)

4. Rectum and Anus

rectum

horizontal fold of
rectum

anal column
(longitudinal fold)

anus

duodenal gland
(gland of Brunner)

small intestine
(jejunum)

villus

teniae coli

semilunar fold of colon

lymphatic
follicle

intestinal
gland

large intestine
(colon)

vermiform
appendix

muco-
epidermis

proper
mucous
membrane

mucous membrane

muscular
layer of
mucosa

submucosa

muscular tunic
of intestine

serosa

61

The Liver

•Length: approx 25 cm, width: approx 15 cm, depth: approx 7 cm, weight: approx 1200–1400 g

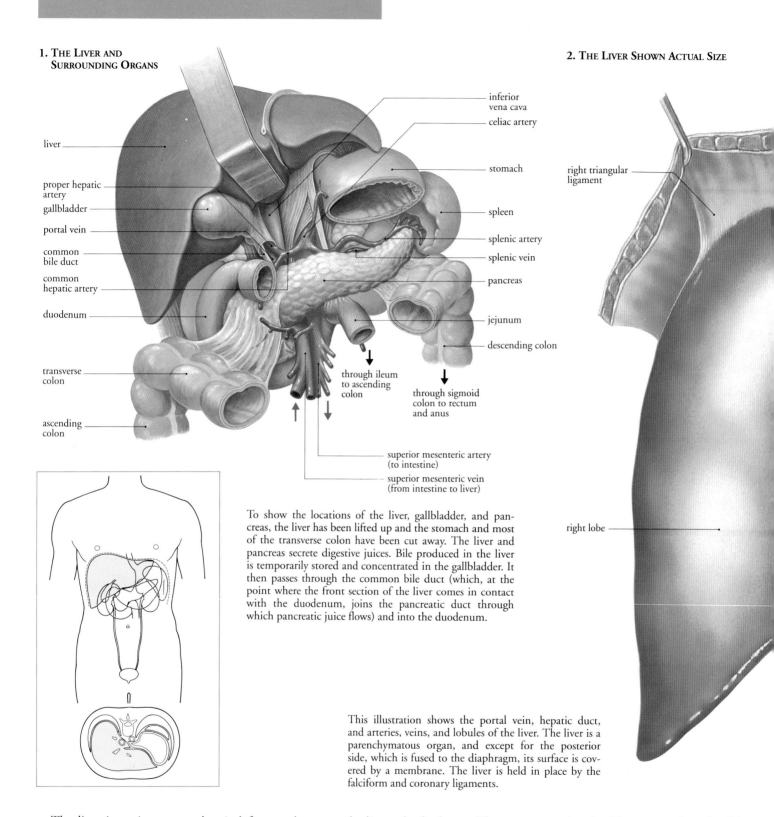

1. THE LIVER AND SURROUNDING ORGANS

2. THE LIVER SHOWN ACTUAL SIZE

liver

proper hepatic artery

gallbladder

portal vein

common bile duct

common hepatic artery

duodenum

transverse colon

ascending colon

inferior vena cava

celiac artery

stomach

spleen

splenic artery

splenic vein

pancreas

jejunum

descending colon

through ileum to ascending colon

through sigmoid colon to rectum and anus

superior mesenteric artery (to intestine)

superior mesenteric vein (from intestine to liver)

right triangular ligament

right lobe

To show the locations of the liver, gallbladder, and pancreas, the liver has been lifted up and the stomach and most of the transverse colon have been cut away. The liver and pancreas secrete digestive juices. Bile produced in the liver is temporarily stored and concentrated in the gallbladder. It then passes through the common bile duct (which, at the point where the front section of the liver comes in contact with the duodenum, joins the pancreatic duct through which pancreatic juice flows) and into the duodenum.

This illustration shows the portal vein, hepatic duct, and arteries, veins, and lobules of the liver. The liver is a parenchymatous organ, and except for the posterior side, which is fused to the diaphragm, its surface is covered by a membrane. The liver is held in place by the falciform and coronary ligaments.

The liver is an important chemical factory that controls diverse functions essential for maintaining life. It produces bile, which aids digestion, and it extracts toxins and synthesizes nutrients that have been absorbed in the blood. When necessary, the liver also adjusts circulating levels of metabolites.

Location. Attached to the lower part of the diaphragm, the liver takes up almost the entire upper right section of the abdominal region, and the upper left section reaches into the thoracic region.

Shape and Size. Viewed from the front, the liver is a right triangle with the hypotenuse facing the tail end (lower side) and the right angle at upper left (the right lobe). The upper side follows the gentle curve of the diaphragm. The part connected to the right upper peritoneal wall is the thickest; the liver becomes thinner and more pointed toward the left.

The liver is the largest organ in the body, weighing approximately 1200–1400 g in the adult. It is heaviest from the ages of 20–40, gradually becoming lighter thereafter. Aside from the section that is attached to the diaphragm, most of the liver is covered by the peritoneum. It is glossy in appearance, and because of the abundance of blood within, it is deep red in color.

Structure. The liver is divided into two parts by the falciform ligament, the right lobe and the left lobe. The left lobe is small, taking up only about one-third to one-sixth of the whole. When

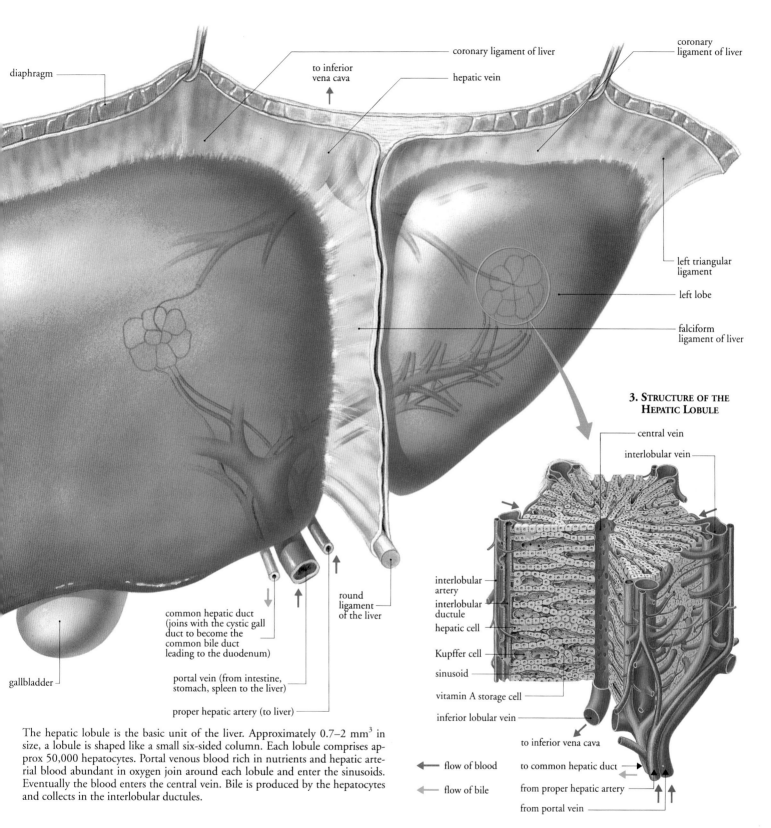

diaphragm

coronary ligament of liver

to inferior vena cava

hepatic vein

coronary ligament of liver

left triangular ligament

left lobe

falciform ligament of liver

3. STRUCTURE OF THE HEPATIC LOBULE

central vein

interlobular vein

interlobular artery

interlobular ductule

hepatic cell

Kupffer cell

sinusoid

vitamin A storage cell

inferior lobular vein

to inferior vena cava

⬅ flow of blood

⬅ flow of bile

to common hepatic duct

from proper hepatic artery

from portal vein

common hepatic duct (joins with the cystic gall duct to become the common bile duct leading to the duodenum)

portal vein (from intestine, stomach, spleen to the liver)

proper hepatic artery (to liver)

round ligament of the liver

gallbladder

The hepatic lobule is the basic unit of the liver. Approximately 0.7–2 mm³ in size, a lobule is shaped like a small six-sided column. Each lobule comprises approx 50,000 hepatocytes. Portal venous blood rich in nutrients and hepatic arterial blood abundant in oxygen join around each lobule and enter the sinusoids. Eventually the blood enters the central vein. Bile is produced by the hepatocytes and collects in the interlobular ductules.

viewed under a microscope, it can be seen that the liver is made of a vast number of units called hepatic lobules. Hepatic lobules are very small, approx 0.7–2 mm³ each, and shaped like closely arranged six-sided pillars or cylinders.

Hepatic Lobules and Blood Vessels. Blood from two vascular systems flows through the basic unit of the liver—the hepatic lobule. One is arterial blood rich in oxygen from the hepatic arteries (common hepatic artery, proper hepatic artery), and the other is venous blood from the portal vein, which leads from the alimentary canal, or digestive tract, and the spleen. This blood is rich in nutrients and other elements. The two types of blood flow are arranged together around the hepatic lobules (interlobular arteries, interlobular veins). After blood has flowed through the tissue of the liver and performed its functions, it flows from the inferior lobular vein to the hepatic vein and the inferior vena cava.

The amount of blood flowing through the adult liver is about 1000–1800 ml per min, 25% of the output of the heart in 1 min. Of this amount, three-fourths to four-fifths comes from the portal vein and the remaining one-fifth comes from the hepatic artery. The amount of blood supplied by the hepatic artery is not large, but the hepatic artery plays an important role as the source of oxygen necessary for the liver to maintain its functions.

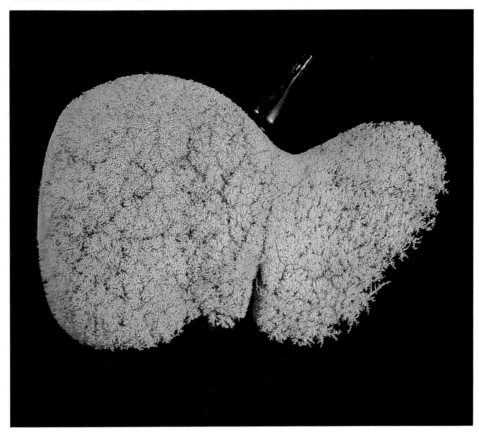

Front view of a model of the liver. The model was constructed by injecting colored plastic into the vascular system of the liver of a normal adult and melting away the liver tissue.

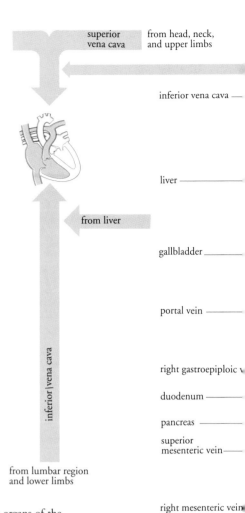

superior vena cava

from head, neck, and upper limbs

inferior vena cava

liver

from liver

gallbladder

portal vein

inferior vena cava

right gastroepiploic v

duodenum

pancreas

superior mesenteric vein

from lumbar region and lower limbs

right mesenteric vein

mesentery

vein of small intestin

ileocolic vein

Oxygen is transported to the various organs of the abdominal region by arteries that branch off the abdominal aorta and nutrients from the digestive tract and hormones are sent to the liver by the portal vein (shown in purple in the diagram), which connects the digestive tract and the liver. After undergoing various chemical processes, the blood returns as venous blood to the hepatic vein and the inferior vena cava to be sent back to the heart.

Functions. The liver has many functions, and its activities are vital to the maintenance of life (for example, it neutralizes harmful toxins transported from the rest of the body). The liver has an ability not found in other organs of regenerating itself: If as much as three-fourths to four-fifths of the organ is removed, it is able to grow back to its original size.

Regulating Metabolism. The liver produces and stores glycogen, a substance that stores energy in order to regulate blood sugar level. The liver synthesizes, dissolves, and stores amino acids, protein, and fat. It stores various vitamins in forms ready for use by the body. The liver also disposes of wastes, such as ammonia and hormones, that are no longer needed by the body. The production and secretion of bile is another of the liver's important functions.

Protecting the Body. The liver breaks down alcohol and other harmful substances, disposing them into bile. It regulates blood volume by storing blood and releasing it as needed. The Kupffer cells, located on the walls of the blood vessels (sinusoids), break down old red blood cells and store iron, a component of hemoglobin. The liver is also involved in the production of antibodies (gamma globulin).

Distribution and Role of the Portal Vein. Veins are widely distributed throughout the digestive tract, and the blood carries various nutrients absorbed in the alimentary canal. These veins converge in the portal vein, which is the blood vessel that transports blood to the great chemical factory that is the liver, where it is assimilated and catabolized.

The portal vein also carries various hormones as well as byproducts from the breakdown of red corpuscles in the spleen to the liver. In the alimentary canal the arteries have divided into a network of capillaries that then become veins that come together at the portal vein where it once more separates into a capillary network. This structure makes the portal vein unique because it has a network of blood capillaries at each end. (Other types of veins have such a network of capillaries only at the end that connects to arteries.)

Major Disorders: hepatitis, cirrhosis, hepatic insufficiency, liver cancer (primary, metastatic), drug-related disorders.

5. DISTRIBUTION OF THE PORTAL VEIN AND BLOOD CIRCULATION

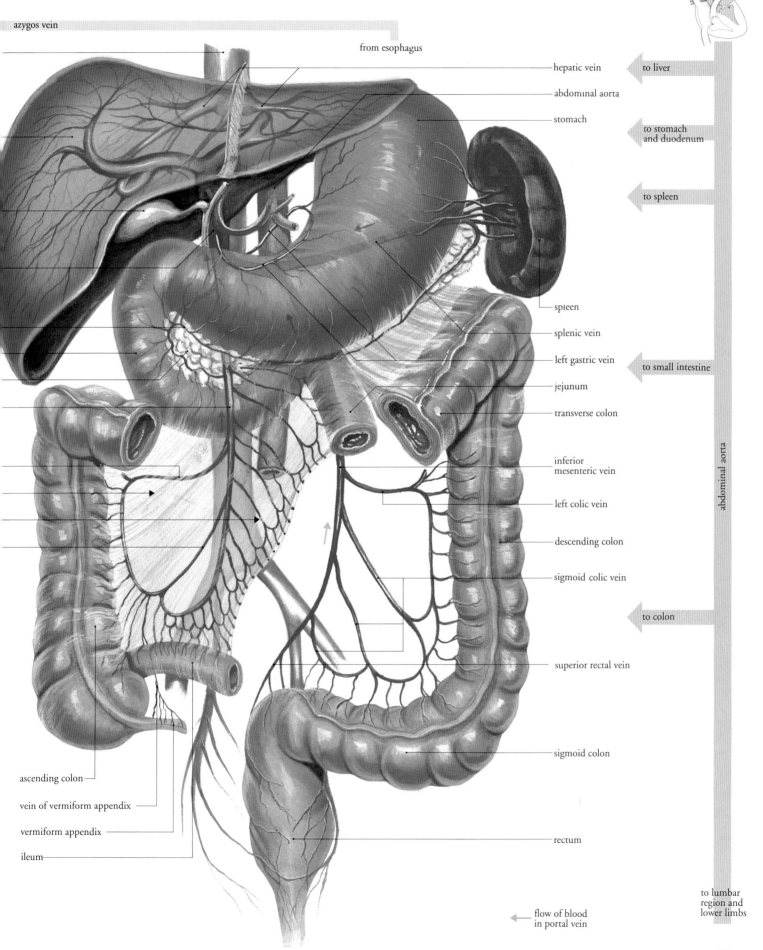

azygos vein

from esophagus

hepatic vein

abdominal aorta

stomach

to liver

to stomach and duodenum

to spleen

spleen

splenic vein

left gastric vein

jejunum

transverse colon

to small intestine

inferior mesenteric vein

left colic vein

descending colon

sigmoid colic vein

to colon

superior rectal vein

sigmoid colon

abdominal aorta

ascending colon

vein of vermiform appendix

vermiform appendix

ileum

rectum

flow of blood in portal vein

to lumbar region and lower limbs

The Gallbladder and Pancreas

- **Gallbladder:** Length: approx 7–9 cm, width: approx 2–3 cm, volume: approx 30–50 ml
- **Pancreas:** Length: approx 15 cm, thickness of the head section: approx 3 cm, weight: approx 70–100 g

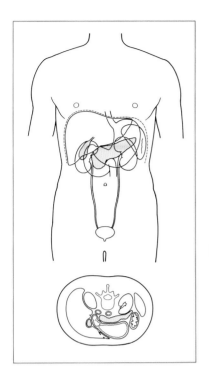

1. THE GALLBLADDER SHOWN ACTUAL SIZE

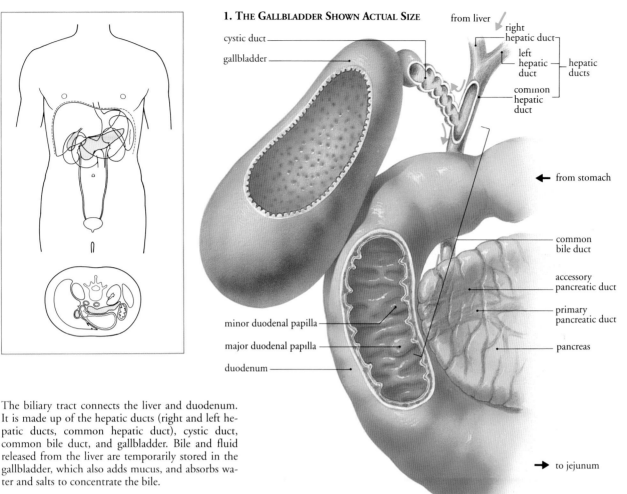

cystic duct

gallbladder

from liver

right hepatic duct

left hepatic duct

common hepatic duct

hepatic ducts

common hepatic arte

proper hepatic artery (to liver)

stomach

from stomach

right gastroepiploic a

right gastroepiploic v

portal vein (to liver)

gastroduodenal arter

common bile duct

accessory pancreatic duct

primary pancreatic duct

pancreas

minor duodenal papilla

major duodenal papilla

duodenum

duodenum

to jejunum

The biliary tract connects the liver and duodenum. It is made up of the hepatic ducts (right and left hepatic ducts, common hepatic duct), cystic duct, common bile duct, and gallbladder. Bile and fluid released from the liver are temporarily stored in the gallbladder, which also adds mucus, and absorbs water and salts to concentrate the bile.

GALLBLADDER

The gallbladder is a small organ located below the liver. It concentrates and stores bile that is produced in the liver.

Location. The gallbladder is attached to a cavity (gallbladder fossa) in the lower section of the liver. From the ventral side a small portion of its tail section is in view.

Shape and Size. Shaped like a pear, the gallbladder is approx 7–9 cm in length, 2–3 cm in width, with a volume of approx 30–50 ml.

Structure. The wall of the gallbladder is composed of mucous membrane packed with numerous folds (mucosal folds), a smooth muscle layer, and a serous covering. It is thin, flexible, and able to stretch considerably. The neck of the gallbladder is attached to the cystic duct, which joins with the hepatic duct from the liver to become the common bile duct that opens into the duodenum.

Function. Approximately half the bile released by the liver is stored in the gallbladder. The bile is then concentrated 1/5 to 1/10 by absorption of water and sodium, mucus is added, and it is combined with food and passed into the duodenum. If food high in fat content is present, amino acids and fatty acids stimulate the duodenum and jejunum to secrete the hormone cholecystokinin. This hormone causes the smooth muscles of the gallbladder to contract and excrete additional bile, which aids in the digestion of fatty materials.

PANCREAS

The pancreas, located behind the stomach, produces strong digestive enzymes. It also secretes insulin and glucagon, which regulate the amount of glucose in blood.

Location. The pancreas is located posterior to the stomach and behind the peritoneum on the ventral side of the first and second lumbar vertebrae. The head section of the pancreas is embraced by the curve of the C-shaped duodenum.

Shape and Size. The pancreas is flat and thin and shaped like a comma. It is thickest (approx 3 cm) and widest at the head section, weighs approx 70–100 g, and is approx 15 cm in length. It is light red and white in color and elastic like rubber.

Structure. The exocrine cells of the pancreas produce pancreatic juice and excrete it to the duodenum. The endocrine cells secrete the hormones insulin (from beta cells) and glucagon (from alpha cells) into the bloodstream. The endocrine cells are distributed like round islands within the exocrine cells and are called pancreatic islets, or islets of Langerhans.

Function. Pancreatic juice includes enzymes that digest protein, fat, and carbohydrates (starch). When the contents of the stomach enter the duodenum, digestive hormones are released from the mucous membrane of the duodenum, stimulating synthesis of digestive enzymes and secretion of pancreatic juice. Insulin promotes use of glucose by the muscles and other tissues, lowering blood sugar level. Glucagon promotes breakdown of glycogen in the pancreas, raising blood sugar level.

Major Disorders: cholecystitis (inflammation of the gallbladder), cancer of the gallbladder, gallstones, pancreatitis, pancreatic cancer, pancreatic lithiasis, diabetes mellitus.

2. THE PANCREAS SHOWN ACTUAL SIZE

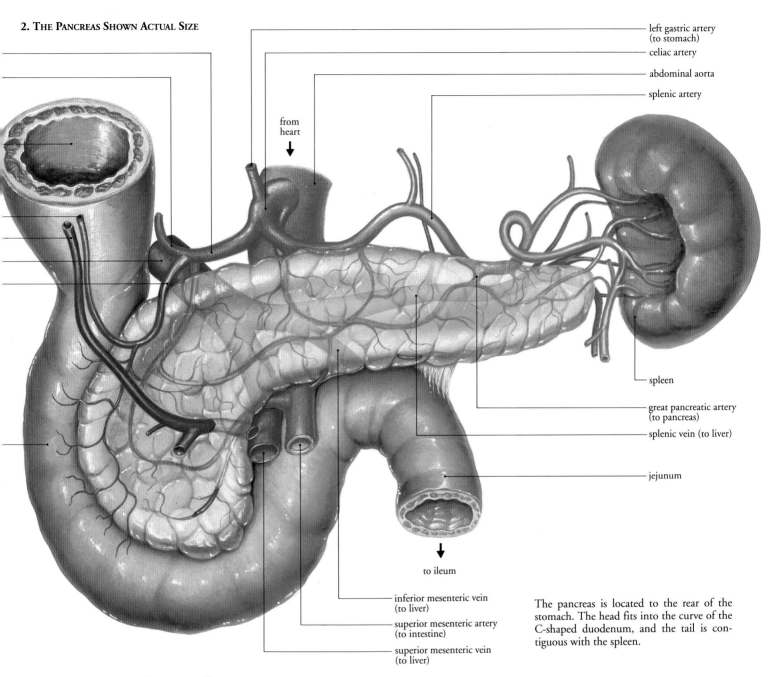

left gastric artery (to stomach)

celiac artery

abdominal aorta

splenic artery

from heart

spleen

great pancreatic artery (to pancreas)

splenic vein (to liver)

jejunum

to ileum

inferior mesenteric vein (to liver)

superior mesenteric artery (to intestine)

superior mesenteric vein (to liver)

The pancreas is located to the rear of the stomach. The head fits into the curve of the C-shaped duodenum, and the tail is contiguous with the spleen.

3. PATH OF PANCREATIC DUCTS AND OUTLETS

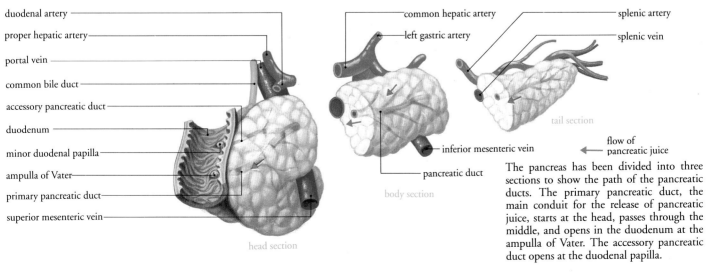

duodenal artery

proper hepatic artery

portal vein

common bile duct

accessory pancreatic duct

duodenum

minor duodenal papilla

ampulla of Vater

primary pancreatic duct

superior mesenteric vein

common hepatic artery

left gastric artery

splenic artery

splenic vein

inferior mesenteric vein

pancreatic duct

body section

tail section

head section

flow of pancreatic juice

The pancreas has been divided into three sections to show the path of the pancreatic ducts. The primary pancreatic duct, the main conduit for the release of pancreatic juice, starts at the head, passes through the middle, and opens in the duodenum at the ampulla of Vater. The accessory pancreatic duct opens at the duodenal papilla.

The Spleen

•Length: approx 10 cm, width: approx 7 cm, thickness: approx 2.5 cm, weight: approx 80–120 g

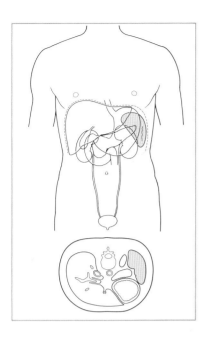

1. The Spleen Shown Actual Size

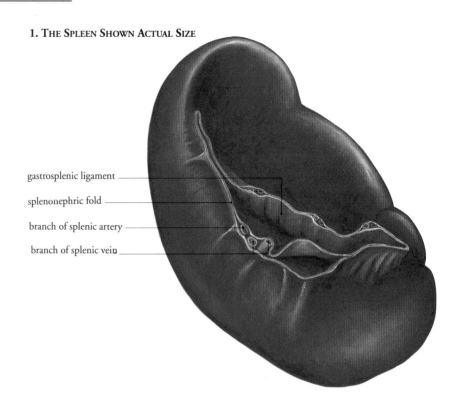

gastrosplenic ligament

splenonephric fold

branch of splenic artery

branch of splenic vein

2. Rear View of Arteries and Veins of the Spleen and Surrounding Organs

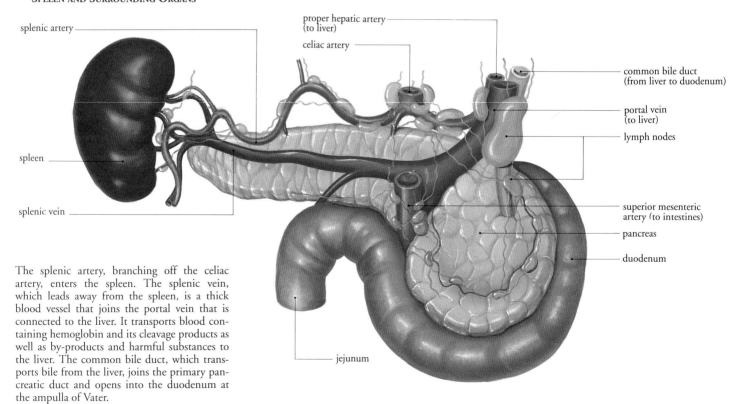

splenic artery

spleen

splenic vein

proper hepatic artery (to liver)

celiac artery

common bile duct (from liver to duodenum)

portal vein (to liver)

lymph nodes

superior mesenteric artery (to intestines)

pancreas

duodenum

jejunum

The splenic artery, branching off the celiac artery, enters the spleen. The splenic vein, which leads away from the spleen, is a thick blood vessel that joins the portal vein that is connected to the liver. It transports blood containing hemoglobin and its cleavage products as well as by-products and harmful substances to the liver. The common bile duct, which transports bile from the liver, joins the primary pancreatic duct and opens into the duodenum at the ampulla of Vater.

The spleen is a lymphatic organ adjacent to the stomach. It breaks down old blood cells and is also involved in the body's immune system.

Location. Located above and posterior to the greater curvature of the stomach, the spleen is contiguous with the tail of the pancreas. The spleen is located in the rear left and closely connected to the inner side of the ninth through eleventh ribs.

Size and Shape. The spleen is dark red and shaped like a broad bean. It is approx 10 cm in length, 2.4 cm thick, and weighs approx 80–120 g. When it becomes enlarged because of disease, it swells up in the direction of the navel and can be palpated in upper left of abdominal region.

Structure. The tunic that covers the spleen extends inside to form a fibrous three-dimensional network of holes (trabeculae). Between the trabeculae are countless white club-shaped nodules (white pulp) buried in red tissue (red pulp). A lattice of fibers (reticular fibers) provides support for the red pulp and is surrounded by cells (reticulocytes). This structure resembles that of lymph nodes (cf., p. 125, Fig. 2) and bone marrow (cf., p. 112, Fig. 1).

Function. An organ of the lymphatic system, the spleen filters blood and destroys old blood cells by sending them to the liver and elsewhere. The spleen also removes foreign matter such as bacteria and produces lymphocytes, cells that are essential for immunity. In humans, the spleen also stores blood to meet additional demands.

Major Disorders: thrombocytopenia (purpura), idiopathic portal hypertension, Banti's syndrome.

The Kidneys

•**Kidney:** Length: approx 11 cm, thickness: approx 5.5 cm, weight: approx 130 g
•**Ureter:** Length: approx 30 cm

1. THE KIDNEY AND NEIGHBORING ORGANS

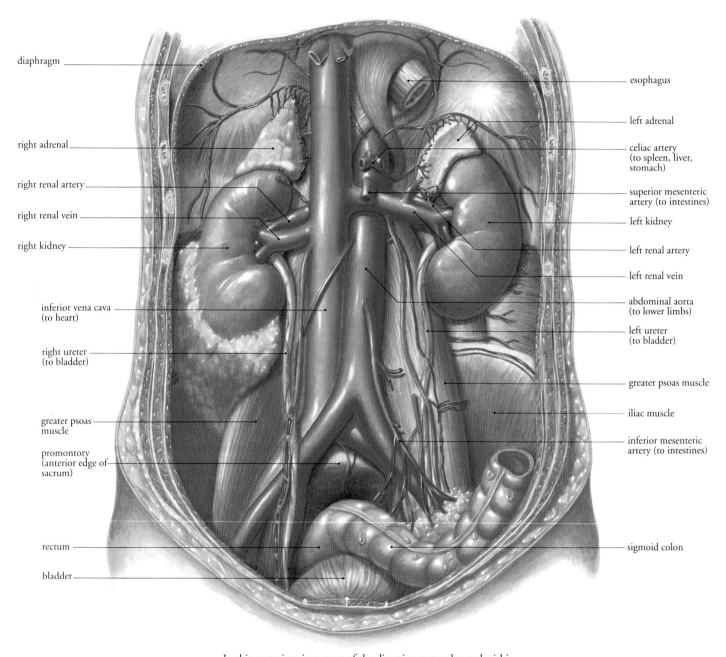

diaphragm

esophagus

left adrenal

right adrenal

celiac artery
(to spleen, liver,
stomach)

right renal artery

superior mesenteric
artery (to intestines)

right renal vein

left kidney

right kidney

left renal artery

left renal vein

inferior vena cava
(to heart)

abdominal aorta
(to lower limbs)

left ureter
(to bladder)

right ureter
(to bladder)

greater psoas muscle

iliac muscle

greater psoas
muscle

inferior mesenteric
artery (to intestines)

promontory
(anterior edge of
sacrum)

rectum

sigmoid colon

bladder

In this posterior view, most of the digestive system located within the peritoneum has been omitted. The kidneys are retroperitoneal organs, i.e., situated to the rear of the peritoneum. The right kidney is positioned slightly lower than the left.

The kidneys are located at about the height of the waist. They filter waste material from the blood and manufacture urine. Hence, the kidneys are the waste treatment center of the body.

Location. The kidneys are retroperitoneal organs—located to the rear of the peritoneum. The left kidney is situated between the eleventh thoracic and third lumbar vertebrae. The right kidney is located slightly lower than the left kidney, because the right lobe of the liver takes up space at its head section.

Size and Shape. Your kidney is slightly larger than your fist. In males the kidney is approx 11 cm long, 5.5 cm thick, and weighs approx 130 g. The kidney is indented on one side, like the kidney bean, and dark red in color.

Structure. A vertical cross section of a kidney shows that the tissue is shaped like a horse's hoof. The hilus, the opening of the hoof, encircles blood vessels, nerves, and the renal pelvis, which is where the ureter enters the kidney. The surface of the kidney is covered by the renal capsule, below this outer layer is the renal cortex, and the medulla is found in the interior. Like a river with multiple tributaries upstream, urine begins its journey in the renal tissue before being transported to the renal papillae. The renal papillae are connected to 7–14 small calyces, which in turn combine to form 2 or 3 large calyces. The urine passes from the large calyces to the renal pelvis in the hilus, where it collects before exiting the kidney via the ureter. The hilus is also the gateway for

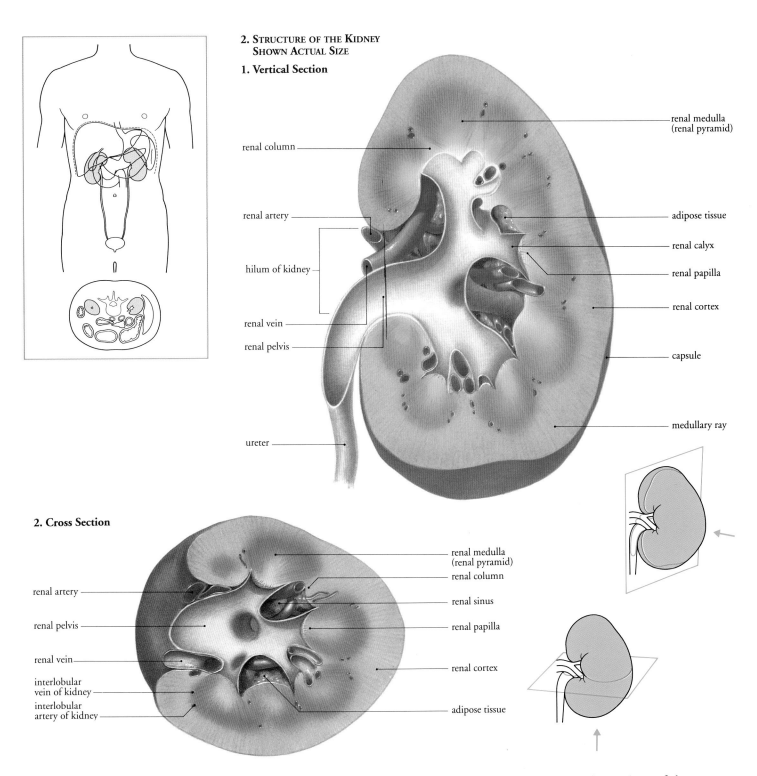

2. STRUCTURE OF THE KIDNEY SHOWN ACTUAL SIZE

1. Vertical Section

renal column

renal artery

hilum of kidney

renal vein

renal pelvis

ureter

renal medulla (renal pyramid)

adipose tissue

renal calyx

renal papilla

renal cortex

capsule

medullary ray

2. Cross Section

renal artery

renal pelvis

renal vein

interlobular vein of kidney

interlobular artery of kidney

renal medulla (renal pyramid)

renal column

renal sinus

renal papilla

renal cortex

adipose tissue

the renal artery (which transports the blood that is the source of urine) and for the renal vein (which transports blood that has been filtered of its waste material).

Function. Blood pumped out by the heart is transported to the kidney to be filtered by the renal glomeruli in the cortex. This blood becomes the raw material for urine (crude urine). The amount of crude urine produced daily is approx 180 l. As the crude urine flows through the renal tubules, which are connected to the glomeruli, dissolved matter (solutes) and water are absorbed once more by the blood. Then part of the matter is excreted by the tubules.

As a result of this complicated process, the urine that is finally excreted from the body amounts to about 1/100 of the amount of crude urine produced, or approx 1.5 l per day. Waste matter and substances ingested in amounts beyond that required by the body are eliminated, whereas proper amounts of matter necessary for body functions (e.g., sugar, sodium) are returned to maintain the necessary elements in blood. For example, in the healthy individual, all the glucose in crude urine is returned to the blood so that almost none is excreted in urine; whereas almost all metabolic waste matter such as urea and creatinine is excreted. If such waste matter is not removed from the blood, serious symptoms of uremic poisoning can develop (e.g., loss of consciousness, convulsions).

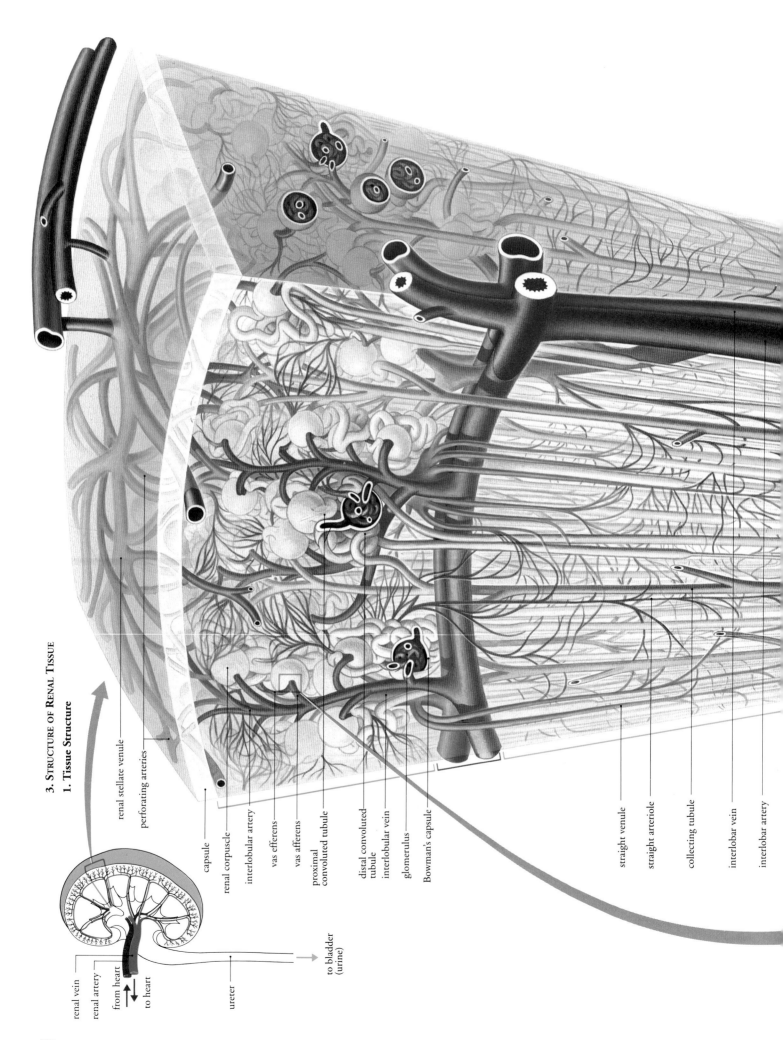

3. STRUCTURE OF RENAL TISSUE

1. Tissue Structure

renal stellate venule

perforating arteries

capsule

renal corpuscle

interlobular artery

vas efferens

vas afferens

proximal
convoluted tubule

distal convoluted
tubule

interlobular vein

glomerulus

Bowman's capsule

straight venule

straight arteriole

collecting tubule

interlobar vein

interlobar artery

renal vein

renal artery

from heart

to heart

ureter

to bladder
(urine)

72

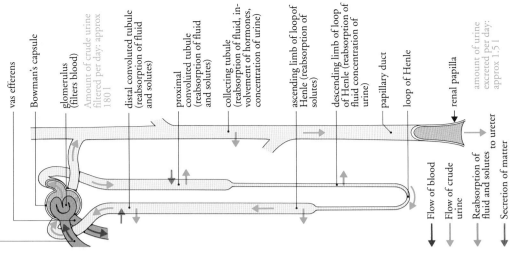

vas afferens
vas efferens
Bowman's capsule
glomerulus (filters blood)
Amount of crude urine filtered per day: approx 180 l
distal convoluted tubule (reabsorption of fluid and solutes)
proximal convoluted tubule (reabsorption of fluid and solutes)
collecting tubule (reabsorption of fluid, involvement of hormones, concentration of urine)
ascending limb of loop of Henle (reabsorption of solutes)
descending limb of loop of Henle (reabsorption of fluid concentration of urine)
papillary duct
loop of Henle
renal papilla
amount of urine excreted per day: approx 1.5 l

Flow of blood
Flow of crude urine
Reabsorption of fluid and solutes
Secretion of matter

to ureter

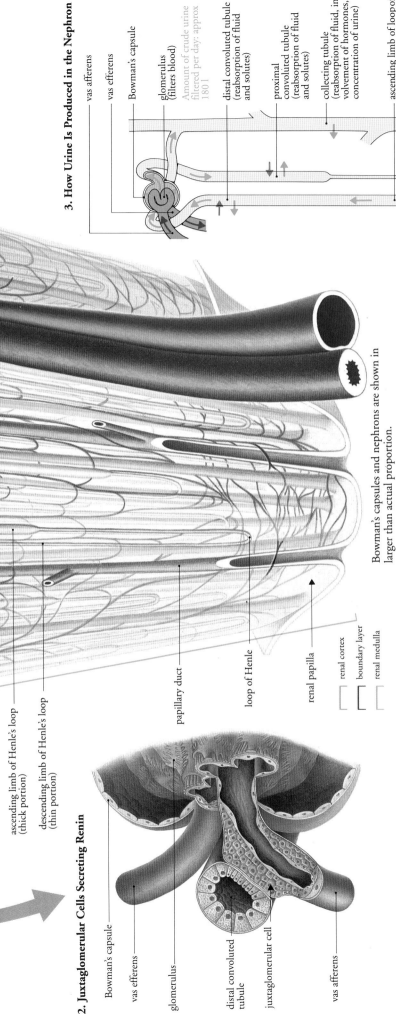

2. Juxtaglomerular Cells Secreting Renin

ascending limb of Henle's loop (thick portion)
descending limb of Henle's loop (thin portion)

papillary duct

loop of Henle

renal papilla

renal cortex
boundary layer
renal medulla

Bowman's capsule
vas efferens
glomerulus
distal convoluted tubule
juxtaglomerular cell
vas afferens

Bowman's capsules and nephrons are shown in larger than actual proportion.

ROLE OF THE KIDNEY

The kidney produces urine and performs the important function of adjusting blood pressure.

How Urine Is Produced. The functional units of the kidney, called nephrons, are made up of glomeruli, which are covered by sacs (Bowman's capsules) and connected to renal tubules. Approximately one million nephrons are found in one human kidney. Individual nephrons cannot be seen by the naked eye. Only vague lines accumulating in the direction of the renal pelvis can be discerned. A renal glomerulus is a filter consisting of thin arteries in a shape resembling a ball of tangled yarn and is approx 0.2 mm in diameter. Filtration is accomplished by blood pressure, which pushes minute particles of matter out through microscopic holes of less than 0.03 μm in diameter (1/250 the diameter of a single red corpuscle).

If the capillaries from both kidneys that make up the glomeruli were stretched in a single line, they would be approx 50 km in length, with total area amounting to approx 1.5 sq m. The crude urine that results from filtering by the glomeruli enters the renal tubules from the Bowman's capsules. One tubule is 10–20 cm in length. The tubules run back and forth through the cortex and medulla in a complex pattern and show variations in thickness and structure, but they do not branch out until after they become collecting tubules.

In the proximal convoluted tubules, the first portion of the renal tubules, 75% of the constituents of crude urine, and 2/3 of the fluid are reabsorbed. At the loop of Henle, the 180° curve of the renal tubule, another 5% of the fluid and sodium are reabsorbed, and by the time the crude urine reaches the beginning of the collecting tubule, 15% of the fluid has been reabsorbed, producing urine. The urine collects in the collecting tubules before passing into the papillary duct and renal calyces to reach the renal pelvis. From the renal pelvis urine passes into the ureter. These complex processes involving fluid and various constituents are regulated by a number of hormones, including aldosterone and antidiuretic hormones.

Regulation of Blood Pressure. An enzyme called renin is secreted by juxtaglomerular cells located in the walls of capillaries in the glomeruli. Renin works on a special protein in blood to produce a substance called angiotensin, which makes the blood vessels contract, raising blood pressure. The kidney also produces substances that lower blood pressure (kallikrein, prostaglandin). These substances work together to maintain blood pressure at normal levels.

Major Disorders: nephritis (glomerulitis), kidney failure, nephrosis, nephropyelitis, kidney stones, hydronephrosis.

The nephron, which is the functional unit of the kidney, consists of small renal bodies (Bowman's capsules and glomeruli) and the connecting renal tubules (proximal convoluted tubules, loop of Henle and distal convoluted tubules, in that order). A single renal tubule can be as long as 10–20 cm. A number of nephrons gather together to form collecting tubules, which eventually become, in turn, the papillary ducts, the renal papillae, and calyces.

The Bladder and Urethra

•**Bladder:** Volume: approx 300–450 ml
•**Urethra:** Length: males approx 16–20 cm, females approx 4–5 cm

1. MALE BLADDER AND URETHRA

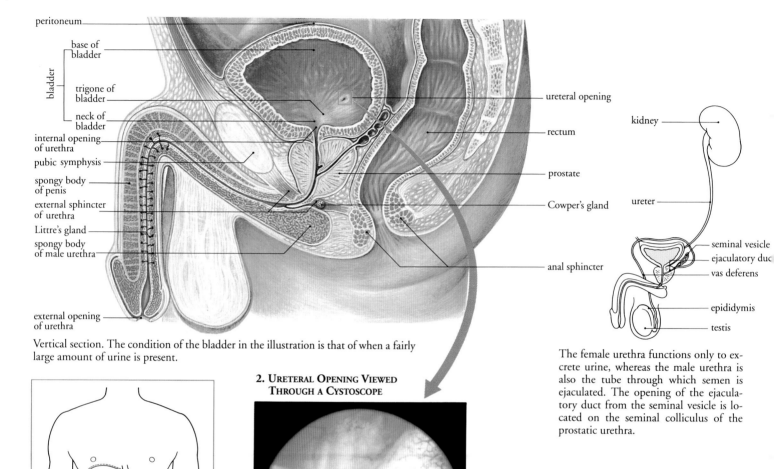

peritoneum
bladder
base of bladder
trigone of bladder
neck of bladder
internal opening of urethra
pubic symphysis
spongy body of penis
external sphincter of urethra
Littre's gland
spongy body of male urethra
external opening of urethra

ureteral opening
rectum
prostate
Cowper's gland
anal sphincter

kidney
ureter
seminal vesicle
ejaculatory duct
vas deferens
epididymis
testis

Vertical section. The condition of the bladder in the illustration is that of when a fairly large amount of urine is present.

The female urethra functions only to excrete urine, whereas the male urethra is also the tube through which semen is ejaculated. The opening of the ejaculatory duct from the seminal vesicle is located on the seminal colliculus of the prostatic urethra.

2. URETERAL OPENING VIEWED THROUGH A CYSTOSCOPE

The ureteral opening seen from within the bladder. The two ureteral ducts of the bladder open and shut at approximately 30-second intervals to release urine into the bladder.

The bladder is a reservoir that temporarily stores urine that has been produced in the kidneys and transported via the ureters. The urethra is the duct that conducts urine from the bladder to be released outside the body.

Location. When the bladder is empty, it remains behind the pubic bone in the pelvis with the peritoneum covering only the head section. As it becomes filled with urine, it begins to swell, becoming round in shape and pushing into the abdominal cavity along the anterior peritoneal wall. The back of the bladder in males is adjacent to the colon; in females it touches the anterior vaginal wall.

In males, the urethra begins at the internal urethral opening and passes through the prostate gland and penis to the external urethral opening. In females it leads straight down from the bladder to the external opening.

Size and Shape. The empty bladder is shaped like a triangle with the base facing upward. It holds approx 300–450 ml of urine. When viewed from the side the urethra in males is S-curved and is 16–20 cm long. In females it is straight and 4–5 cm long.

Structure. The innermost layers of the bladder consists of mucous membrane and submucosa through which pass blood vessels, lymphatic vessels, and nerves. The submucosa is followed by an inner layer of longitudinal muscle, a layer of circular muscle, and an outer layer of longitudinal muscle (all these are smooth muscles). The bladder is covered by an external tunic. The urethra is formed by an inner layer of longitudinal muscle and an outer layer of circular muscle.

Function. The bladder is a reservoir that stores urine until it is voided. Normally, when the urine volume reaches 250 ml or more, the internal pressure reaches its limit (sufficient to produce a column of water of 15–20 cm), and urination must occur. The impulse to urinate arises in response to expansion of the bladder wall and stimulation from the urethra. The sphincter of the urethra relaxes, and the bladder muscles contract to force out urine. This reaction also involves the central nervous system, including the cerebral cortex, brain stem, and hypothalamus.

Major Disorders: cystitis, urinary bladder tumor, vesical diverticulum, prolapse of the bladder, vesicolithiasis, cord bladder, urethritis, urethrophyma, urethral stone.

3. FEMALE BLADDER AND URETHRA

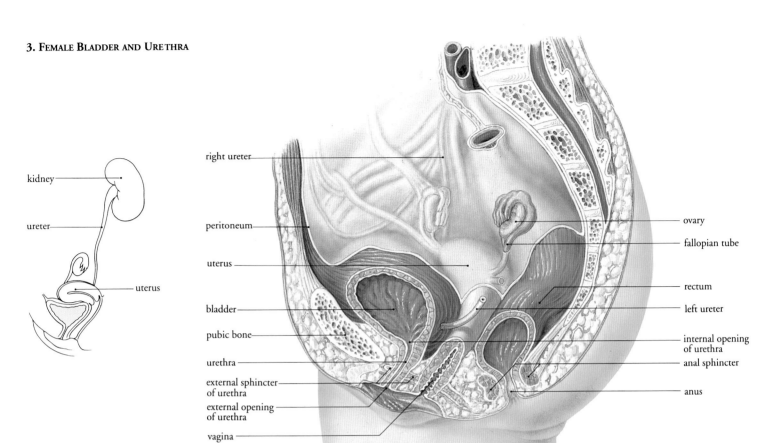

kidney

ureter

uterus

right ureter

peritoneum

uterus

bladder

pubic bone

urethra

external sphincter of urethra

external opening of urethra

vagina

ovary

fallopian tube

rectum

left ureter

internal opening of urethra

anal sphincter

anus

Lateral view. When the bladder is empty it is shaped like a wine glass, as seen in the illustration at left.

The Male Reproductive Organs

•**Penis:** Length: approx 8 cm (at rest)
•**Testis (Testicle):** Length: approx 4–5 cm
•**Seminal Vesicle:** Length: approx 5 cm, width: approx 2 cm, thickness: approx 1 cm
•**Prostate Gland:** Length: approx 2.5 cm, width: approx 4 cm, thickness: approx 1.5 cm, weight: approx 20 g

1. LOCATION OF MALE REPRODUCTIVE ORGANS

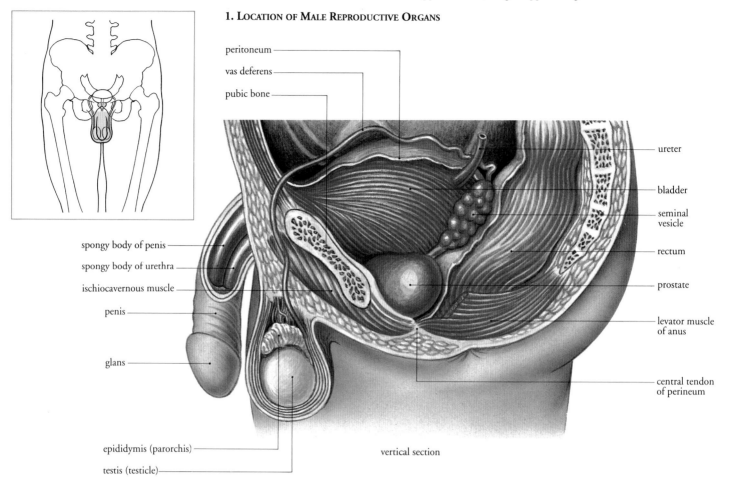

peritoneum
vas deferens
pubic bone

ureter
bladder
seminal vesicle
rectum
prostate
levator muscle of anus
central tendon of perineum

spongy body of penis
spongy body of urethra
ischiocavernous muscle
penis
glans
epididymis (parorchis)
testis (testicle)

vertical section

The male reproductive organs produce spermatozoa, the male reproductive cells, and are used for sexual intercourse. They are made up of internal and external organs. The internal organs include the testes (testicles), epididymis, vas deferens, seminal vesicles, ejaculatory ducts, and the prostate gland. The external organs include the penis and scrotum.

Location. The penis is affixed by its root to the triangular section formed by the left and right ischiopubic rami. It extends down from the pubic symphysis and protrudes outside the body. The scrotum, which houses the testes and epididymides, hangs behind the penis.

The epididymis is situated on top of the testis, and the vas deferens leading from the epididymis passes through the groin into the pelvis and from there through the peritoneum and into the abdominal cavity. After the vas deferens reaches the lower left region of the bladder, it widens to become the ampulla of vas deferens, enters the prostate gland, and becomes the ejaculatory duct. Each ejaculatory duct opens separately into the left and right side of the urethra. The two seminal vesicles, which are long and narrow and shaped like spindles, are behind and below the bladder and above and behind the prostate gland. The ejaculatory ducts open out from these vesicles.

Structure and Function. TESTES. The testis is approx 4–5 cm in length and shaped somewhat like a flat egg. In the first stages of fetal development, the testes grow near the kidneys before descending gradually, and by the time of birth, are enclosed in the scrotum. Wound within each testis are approx 1000 convoluted seminiferous tubules, each of which is almost 1 m in length when stretched out. These tubules begin to produce spermatozoa at pu-

berty. Spermatozoa are transported to the epididymis through the straight tubules. The interstitial tissue filling the space between the seminiferous tubules contains interstitial cells that secrete the male hormone testosterone.

EPIDIDYMIS. The epididymis is a twisted mass of long ducts, each of which is as long as 6 m when stretched out. The spermatozoa from the testis are stored here for 10–20 d.

PENIS. The average length of the penis at rest is about 8 cm. The penis consists of a cylindrical shaft and the glans at the tip. The shaft of the penis is formed by the corpora cavernosa in the back and a spongy structure called the corpus spongiosum toward the end. Each of these bodies is covered by a white membrane. The urethra passes through the length of the penis, and the external opening is at the end of the glans. The bodies of the penis are made of countless trabeculae that crisscross like a net as well as spaces (venous cavities). When blood from the branches of the central artery of the penis fills these venous cavities, the penis swells. This is how an erection occurs.

SEMINAL VESICLE. In the adult male the seminal vesicle is a sac with a volume of about 10–15 cm^3. The interior is divided into numerous small chambers. The seminal vesicles produce a fluid called semen that facilitates the mobility of sperm.

PROSTATE GLAND. The prostate gland weighs approx 20 g in the adult male and is shaped like a walnut. The urethra passes through the center toward the front, and the ejaculatory duct enters diagonally and meets the urethra. This gland secretes a fluid that aids the mobility of sperm. This fluid is part of semen.

Major Disorders: sexually transmitted diseases, prostatomegaly, prostate cancer, oscheohydrocele, phimosis, impotence.

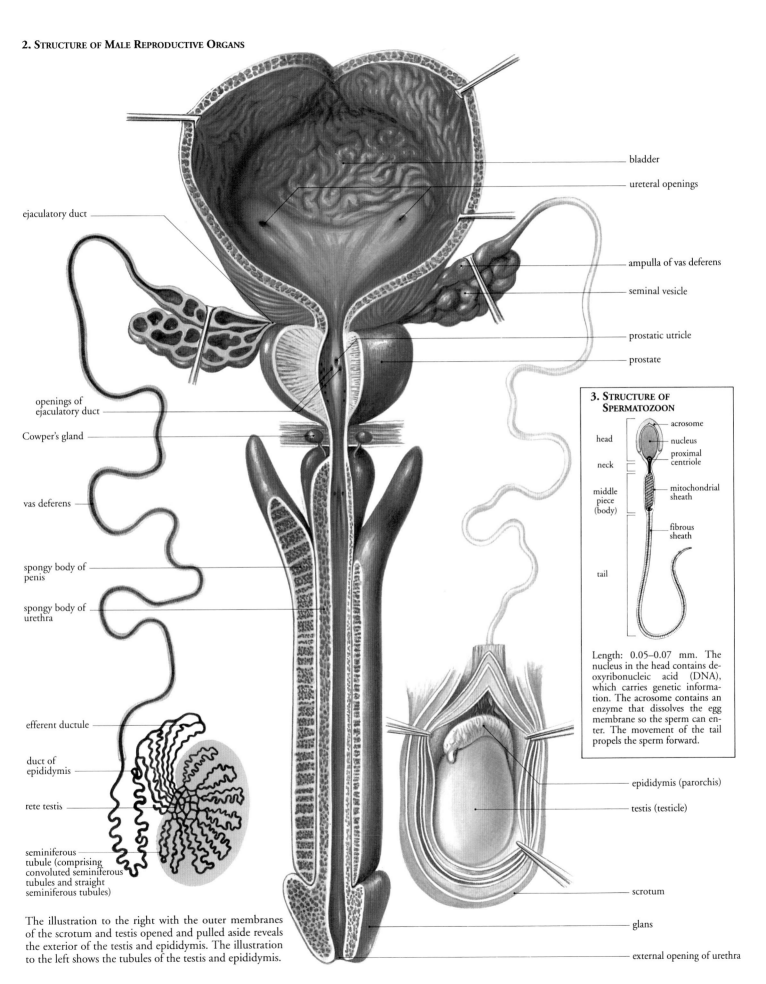

bladder

ureteral openings

ejaculatory duct

ampulla of vas deferens

seminal vesicle

prostatic utricle

prostate

openings of
ejaculatory duct

Cowper's gland

vas deferens

spongy body of
penis

spongy body of
urethra

efferent ductule

duct of
epididymis

rete testis

seminiferous
tubule (comprising
convoluted seminiferous
tubules and straight
seminiferous tubules)

epididymis (parorchis)

testis (testicle)

scrotum

glans

external opening of urethra

3. STRUCTURE OF SPERMATOZOON

head

neck

middle
piece
(body)

tail

acrosome

nucleus

proximal
centriole

mitochondrial
sheath

fibrous
sheath

Length: 0.05–0.07 mm. The nucleus in the head contains deoxyribonucleic acid (DNA), which carries genetic information. The acrosome contains an enzyme that dissolves the egg membrane so the sperm can enter. The movement of the tail propels the sperm forward.

The illustration to the right with the outer membranes of the scrotum and testis opened and pulled aside reveals the exterior of the testis and epididymis. The illustration to the left shows the tubules of the testis and epididymis.

The Female Reproductive Organs

- **Uterus:** Length: approx 7 cm, maximum width: approx 4 cm, thickness: approx 2.5 cm (in the nonpregnant adult female)
- **Fallopian Tube:** Length: approx 10–12 cm
- **Ovary:** Length: approx 2.5–4.0 cm, width: approx 1.2–2.0, thickness: approx 1 cm
- **Vagina:** Length: approx 10 cm

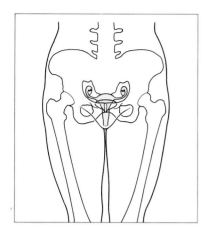

2. LIGAMENTS THAT HOLD THE UTERUS

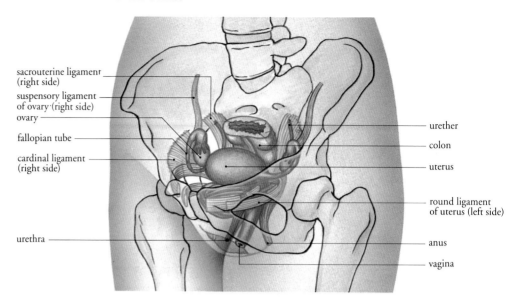

sacrouterine ligament (right side)
suspensory ligament of ovary (right side)
ovary
fallopian tube
cardinal ligament (right side)
urethra

urether
colon
uterus
round ligament of uterus (left side)
anus
vagina

1. LOCATION OF FEMALE REPRODUCTIVE ORGANS

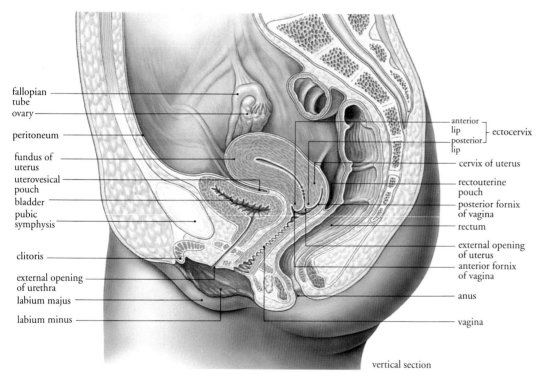

fallopian tube
ovary
peritoneum
fundus of uterus
uterovesical pouch
bladder
pubic symphysis
clitoris
external opening of urethra
labium majus
labium minus

anterior lip
posterior lip
} ectocervix
cervix of uterus
rectouterine pouch
posterior fornix of vagina
rectum
external opening of uterus
anterior fornix of vagina
anus
vagina

vertical section

5. POSTERIOR VIEW OF INTERNAL REPRODUCTIVE ORGANS SHOWN ACTUAL SIZE

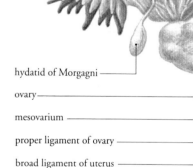

fallopian tube
hydatid of Morgagni
ovary
mesovarium
proper ligament of ovary
broad ligament of uterus

The female reproductive organs are responsible for the production of eggs, the female reproductive cells and, after fertilization, they are involved in the development and birth of the fetus—essential for survival of the species. They are classified into internal and external organs.

INTERNAL REPRODUCTIVE ORGANS— UTERUS, FALLOPIAN TUBES, OVARIES, VAGINA

UTERUS. The uterus leans forward over the bladder ventral to the colon in the pelvis. It resembles an eggplant and is somewhat flattened front and back. The rounded head section is the body of the uterus and the narrow cylindrical tail portion is the cervix. A verticle cross-section of the interior of the uterus shows that it is shaped like a cocktail glass. The openings to the fallopian tubes are found at the upper corners and the isthmus corresponds to the stem of the cocktail glass. The smooth muscle of the uterus is over 1 cm thick. The inner surface is lined by mucous membrane. For the most part, longitudinal muscle fibers ring the uterus. To protect it from tearing when it becomes enlarged during pregnancy, these are reinforced by intersecting fibers. The membrane of the uterus peels away in the course of the menstrual cycle. The mucous membrane of the cervix, however, does not peel away, and it secretes alkaline mucus to prevent infection from entering the uterus from the vagina.

FALLOPIAN TUBES. The fallopian tubes, which resemble earthworms, extend outward from two openings on the left and right side of the uterus. The tubes are approx 10–20 cm in length. At the outer end, the fallopian tube widens to form the ampulla. The distal part of the fallopian tube diverges into numerous

3. Parts of the Female Reproductive Organs

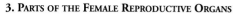

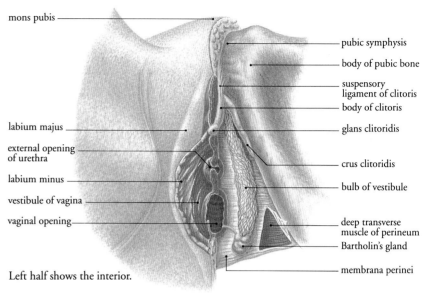

fallopian tube

ampulla of fallopian tube / isthmus of fallopian tube

body of uterus

uterus

cervix of uterus

ovary

labium majus

glans clitoridis

external opening of urethra

vestibule of vagina

labium minus

vaginal opening

external genitalia

internal genitalia

vagina

4. Structure of External Reproductive Organs

mons pubis

pubic symphysis

body of pubic bone

suspensory ligament of clitoris

body of clitoris

labium majus

glans clitoridis

external opening of urethra

crus clitoridis

labium minus

bulb of vestibule

vestibule of vagina

vaginal opening

deep transverse muscle of perineum

Bartholin's gland

membrana perinei

Left half shows the interior.

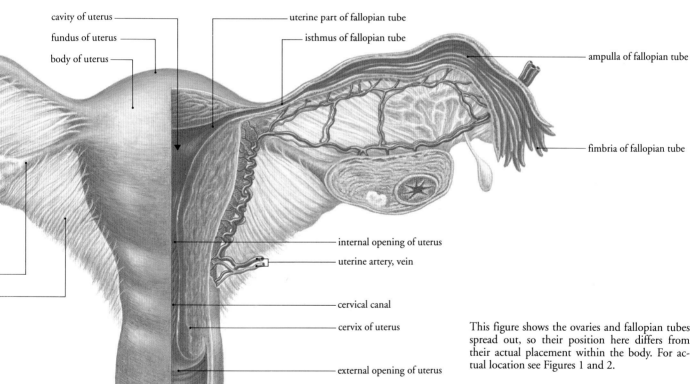

cavity of uterus

uterine part of fallopian tube

fundus of uterus

isthmus of fallopian tube

body of uterus

ampulla of fallopian tube

fimbria of fallopian tube

internal opening of uterus

uterine artery, vein

cervical canal

cervix of uterus

external opening of uterus

vagina

This figure shows the ovaries and fallopian tubes spread out, so their position here differs from their actual placement within the body. For actual location see Figures 1 and 2.

finger-like projections facing the ovary called fimbriae.

OVARIES. The ovaries lie adjacent to the lateral walls of the pelvis, just below the fallopian tubes. (For size, structure, and function, see page 81.)

VAGINA. The vagina is the muscular canal connecting the cervix of the uterus to the vulva. It is about 10 cm long and located between the urethra and the rectum. It is usually narrow because of folds in the mucous membrane (rugae), but can expand considerably. The vagina is acidic to help prevent infection.

EXTERNAL REPRODUCTIVE ORGANS—
CLITORIS, VESTIBULE OF VAGINA, LABIA MINORA, LABIA MAJORA

The labia minora surround the clitoris on the left and right. These are covered by the labia majora. The external urethral open-

ing is located on the ventral side of the vestibule of the vagina and the vaginal opening is posterior to the uretha. The hymen is a membranous fold that may be between the vaginal opening and the vestibule.

The clitoris is homologous to the penis of the male and the labia minora are homologous to the skin of the penis. The labia minora contain no sweat glands, but they are rich in the pigment melanin. The labia majora are homologous to the scrotum of the male. They are thick folds of skin made up primarily of subcutaneous fatty tissue. Bartholin's glands (greater vestibular glands) and the lesser vestibular glands are found in the vestibule of the vagina. These glands secrete mucus.

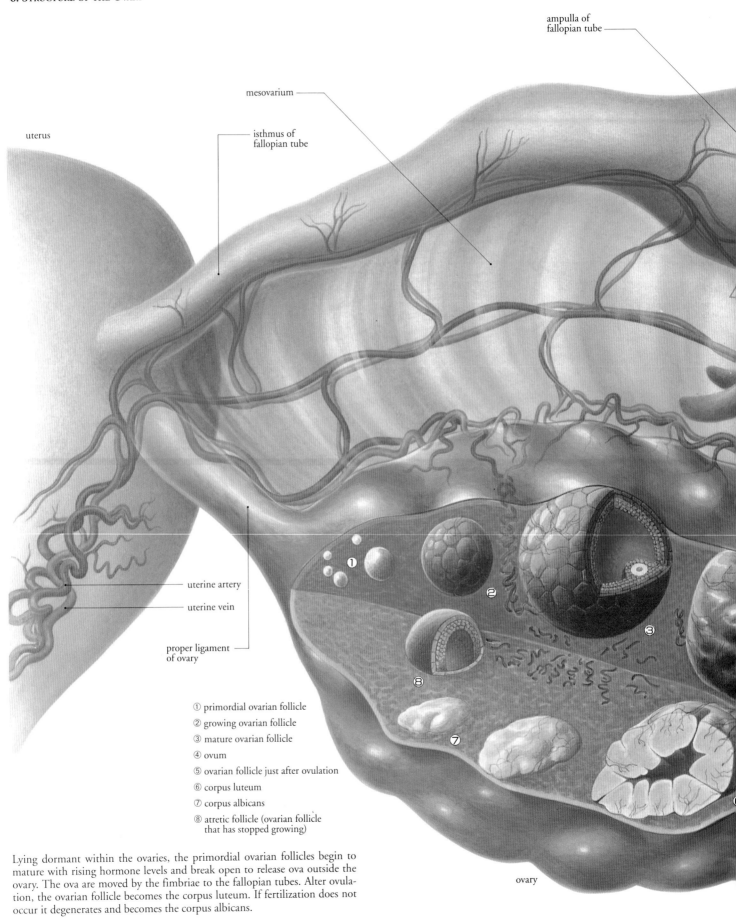

ampulla of
fallopian tube

mesovarium

isthmus of
fallopian tube

uterus

uterine artery

uterine vein

proper ligament
of ovary

① primordial ovarian follicle

② growing ovarian follicle

③ mature ovarian follicle

④ ovum

⑤ ovarian follicle just after ovulation

⑥ corpus luteum

⑦ corpus albicans

⑧ atretic follicle (ovarian follicle
that has stopped growing)

ovary

Lying dormant within the ovaries, the primordial ovarian follicles begin to
mature with rising hormone levels and break open to release ova outside the
ovary. The ova are moved by the fimbriae to the fallopian tubes. Alter ovulation, the ovarian follicle becomes the corpus luteum. If fertilization does not
occur it degenerates and becomes the corpus albicans.

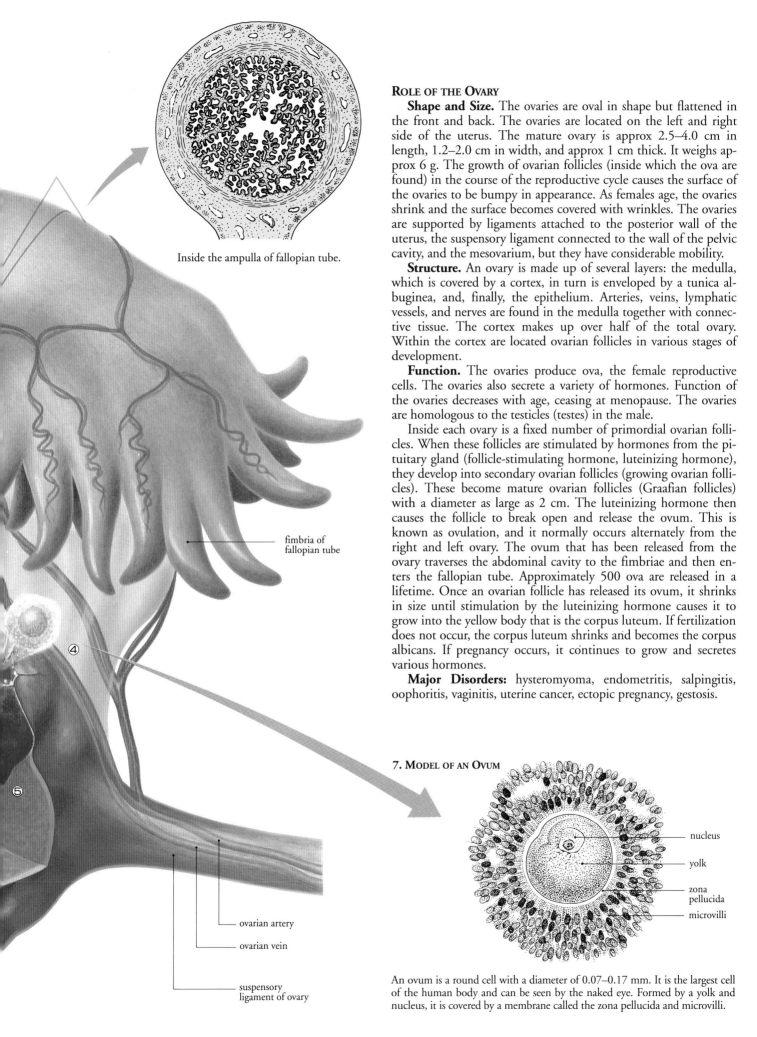

Inside the ampulla of fallopian tube.

fimbria of
fallopian tube

④

⑤

ovarian artery

ovarian vein

suspensory
ligament of ovary

ROLE OF THE OVARY

Shape and Size. The ovaries are oval in shape but flattened in the front and back. The ovaries are located on the left and right side of the uterus. The mature ovary is approx 2.5–4.0 cm in length, 1.2–2.0 cm in width, and approx 1 cm thick. It weighs approx 6 g. The growth of ovarian follicles (inside which the ova are found) in the course of the reproductive cycle causes the surface of the ovaries to be bumpy in appearance. As females age, the ovaries shrink and the surface becomes covered with wrinkles. The ovaries are supported by ligaments attached to the posterior wall of the uterus, the suspensory ligament connected to the wall of the pelvic cavity, and the mesovarium, but they have considerable mobility.

Structure. An ovary is made up of several layers: the medulla, which is covered by a cortex, in turn is enveloped by a tunica albuginea, and, finally, the epithelium. Arteries, veins, lymphatic vessels, and nerves are found in the medulla together with connective tissue. The cortex makes up over half of the total ovary. Within the cortex are located ovarian follicles in various stages of development.

Function. The ovaries produce ova, the female reproductive cells. The ovaries also secrete a variety of hormones. Function of the ovaries decreases with age, ceasing at menopause. The ovaries are homologous to the testicles (testes) in the male.

Inside each ovary is a fixed number of primordial ovarian follicles. When these follicles are stimulated by hormones from the pituitary gland (follicle-stimulating hormone, luteinizing hormone), they develop into secondary ovarian follicles (growing ovarian follicles). These become mature ovarian follicles (Graafian follicles) with a diameter as large as 2 cm. The luteinizing hormone then causes the follicle to break open and release the ovum. This is known as ovulation, and it normally occurs alternately from the right and left ovary. The ovum that has been released from the ovary traverses the abdominal cavity to the fimbriae and then enters the fallopian tube. Approximately 500 ova are released in a lifetime. Once an ovarian follicle has released its ovum, it shrinks in size until stimulation by the luteinizing hormone causes it to grow into the yellow body that is the corpus luteum. If fertilization does not occur, the corpus luteum shrinks and becomes the corpus albicans. If pregnancy occurs, it continues to grow and secretes various hormones.

Major Disorders: hysteromyoma, endometritis, salpingitis, oophoritis, vaginitis, uterine cancer, ectopic pregnancy, gestosis.

7. MODEL OF AN OVUM

nucleus

yolk

zona pellucida

microvilli

An ovum is a round cell with a diameter of 0.07–0.17 mm. It is the largest cell of the human body and can be seen by the naked eye. Formed by a yolk and nucleus, it is covered by a membrane called the zona pellucida and microvilli.

The Mechanism of Menstruation

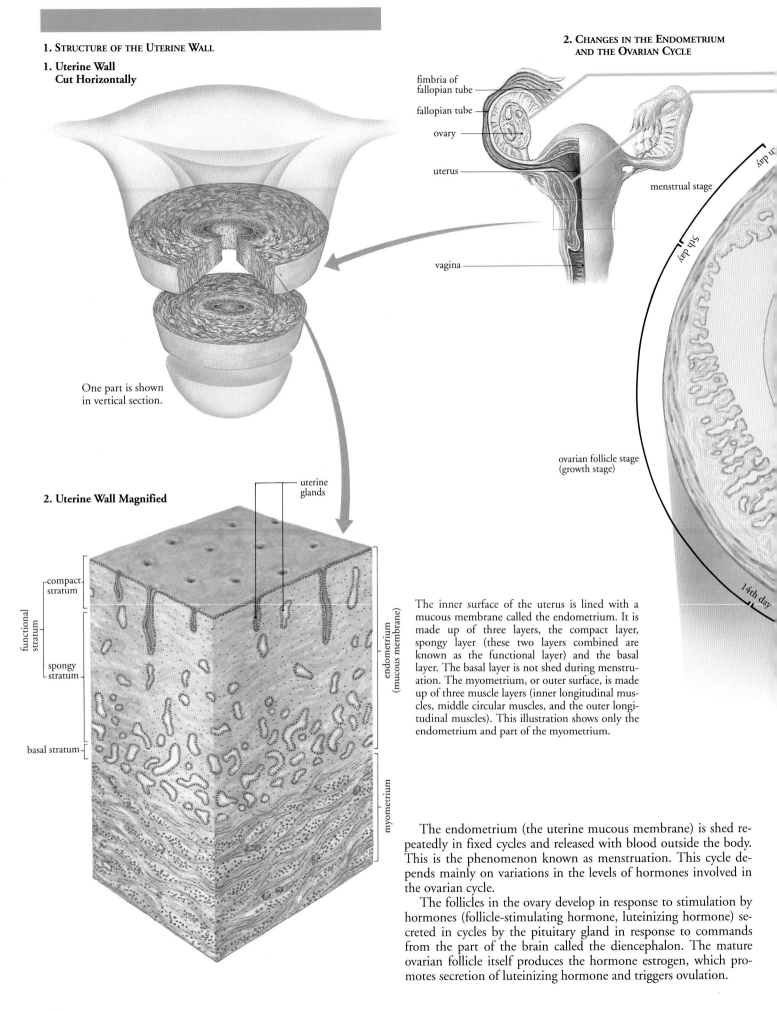

1. STRUCTURE OF THE UTERINE WALL

1. Uterine Wall
Cut Horizontally

One part is shown
in vertical section.

2. Uterine Wall Magnified

uterine
glands

compact
stratum

functional
stratum

spongy
stratum

basal stratum

endometrium
(mucous membrane)

myometrium

2. CHANGES IN THE ENDOMETRIUM AND THE OVARIAN CYCLE

fimbria of
fallopian tube

fallopian tube

ovary

uterus

vagina

menstrual stage

ovarian follicle stage
(growth stage)

11th day

5th day

14th day

The inner surface of the uterus is lined with a mucous membrane called the endometrium. It is made up of three layers, the compact layer, spongy layer (these two layers combined are known as the functional layer) and the basal layer. The basal layer is not shed during menstruation. The myometrium, or outer surface, is made up of three muscle layers (inner longitudinal muscles, middle circular muscles, and the outer longitudinal muscles). This illustration shows only the endometrium and part of the myometrium.

The endometrium (the uterine mucous membrane) is shed repeatedly in fixed cycles and released with blood outside the body. This is the phenomenon known as menstruation. This cycle depends mainly on variations in the levels of hormones involved in the ovarian cycle.

The follicles in the ovary develop in response to stimulation by hormones (follicle-stimulating hormone, luteinizing hormone) secreted in cycles by the pituitary gland in response to commands from the part of the brain called the diencephalon. The mature ovarian follicle itself produces the hormone estrogen, which promotes secretion of luteinizing hormone and triggers ovulation.

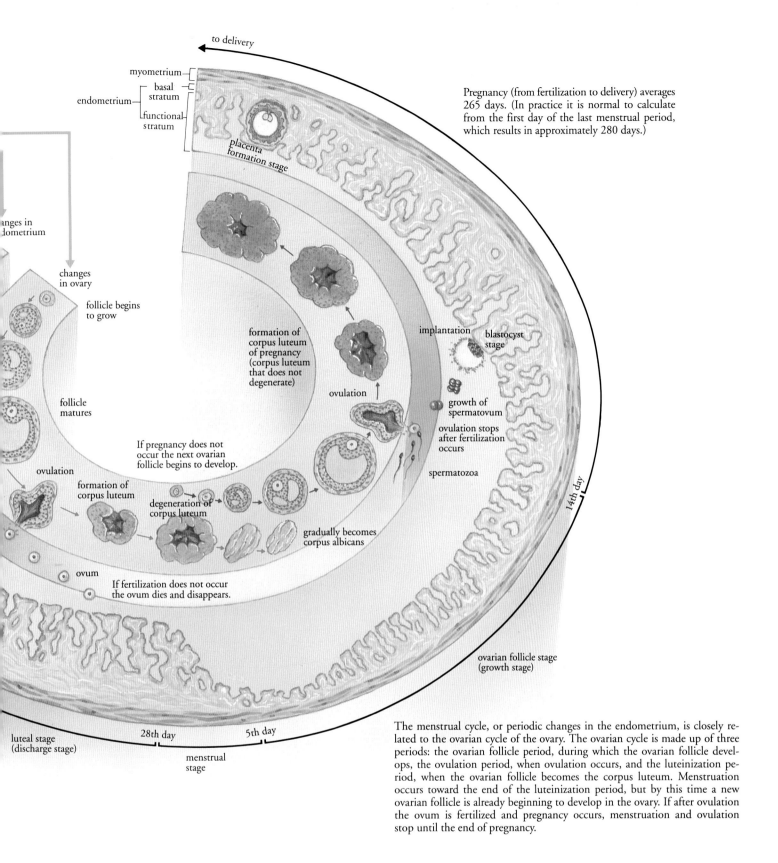

to delivery

myometrium
basal stratum
endometrium
functional stratum

placenta formation stage

Pregnancy (from fertilization to delivery) averages 265 days. (In practice it is normal to calculate from the first day of the last menstrual period, which results in approximately 280 days.)

...anges in ...dometrium

changes in ovary

follicle begins to grow

formation of corpus luteum of pregnancy (corpus luteum that does not degenerate)

follicle matures

ovulation

implantation

blastocyst stage

follicle

If pregnancy does not occur the next ovarian follicle begins to develop.

ovulation

formation of corpus luteum

degeneration of corpus luteum

growth of spermatovum

ovulation stops after fertilization occurs

spermatozoa

14th day

gradually becomes corpus albicans

ovum

If fertilization does not occur the ovum dies and disappears.

ovarian follicle stage (growth stage)

luteal stage (discharge stage)

28th day

5th day

menstrual stage

The menstrual cycle, or periodic changes in the endometrium, is closely related to the ovarian cycle of the ovary. The ovarian cycle is made up of three periods: the ovarian follicle period, during which the ovarian follicle develops, the ovulation period, when ovulation occurs, and the luteinization period, when the ovarian follicle becomes the corpus luteum. Menstruation occurs toward the end of the luteinization period, but by this time a new ovarian follicle is already beginning to develop in the ovary. If after ovulation the ovum is fertilized and pregnancy occurs, menstruation and ovulation stop until the end of pregnancy.

Follicles that remain in the ovary after the release of an ovum become corpus luteum, which secrete luteinizing hormone (progesterone). The ovum enters the fallopian tube, and if it is not fertilized, it dies and is absorbed by the body. The corpus luteum then withers and becomes corpus albicans, and secretion of luteinizing hormone rapidly diminishes.

The surface of the endometrium continues to grow and develop as long as hormones from the ovary (estrogen, progesterone) are being secreted, but when secretion declines, changes occur in the special vascular system of the functional layer of the endometrium, stopping the blood supply and inducing necrosis of the functional layer, which then peels away. These characteristic blood vessels are not present in the basal layer so it does not react to changes in hormone levels and consequently does not peel off. Over a period of about one month this functional layer grows again with the increase in hormone levels.

The normal ovulation cycle is every 28–30 d. The normal menstrual cycle (from the first day of one menstrual period to the first day of the next) is about 25–38 d. The normal level of menstrual blood flow varies 20–120 ml, with an average of approx 50 ml.

Pregnancy

From Fertilization to Implantation. Sperm that has been ejaculated during sexual intercourse moves at a speed of 2–3 mm per minute through the vagina, cervix, uterus, and into the fallopian tube. It takes approx 3–15 hr for the sperm to reach the ampulla of the fallopian tube where it encounters the ovum. After ovulation, the ovum is caught by the fimbriae of the fallopian tube and transported to the ampulla where it encounters the sperm. Sperm is capable of fertiliziation from 30 hr to 3 d after ejaculation, and the ovum can be fertilized for 24 hr after ovulation.

The fertilized egg divides and multiplies, and as it grows it is transported by the movement of the microvilli and the undulating movement of the wall of the fallopian tube to the uterus, a journey that takes approx 3–4 d. In the uterus, new blood vessels have formed and the fertilized ovum is implanted on the endometrium, which is secreting mucus. It takes 6 d from fertilization to implantation. By the time the ovum enters the uterus, it is a collection of 64–128 cells, and at implantation it has a central cavity and is called a blastula.

Formation of the Placenta. A short while after the fertilized ovum has become implanted on the endometrium, the placenta forms from both the ovum and the endometrium. Formation of the placenta begins about the 5th wk after fertilization and is completed by the 13th wk; it continues to grow until about the 8th mo of pregnancy.

The placenta receives the oxygen and nutrients necessary for the fetus to grow from the blood of the mother. The placenta also secretes various hormones necessary for a normal pregnancy. The placenta is a circular spongy organ with numerous blood vessels, and at the end of pregnancy it weighs approx 500 g, has a diameter of approx 15–20 cm and is about 1.5–3.0 cm thick.

Expansion of the Uterus. The uterus of the nonpregnant woman fits within the small pelvic cavity. It is 7 cm long and weighs 40–65 g. The uterus of a pregnant woman begins to protrude into the abdominal cavity and the base begins to touch the ventral abdominal wall by the 4th mo of pregnancy. By the end of the pregnancy it is about 36 cm long and weighs as much as 1 kg. In just over 9 mo the space within the uterus enlarges by 2000–2500 times, occupying a large part of the abdominal region.

Major Disorders: extrauterine pregnancy, hydatid mole, placenta previa.

1. Changes in the Ovum from Fertilization to Implantation

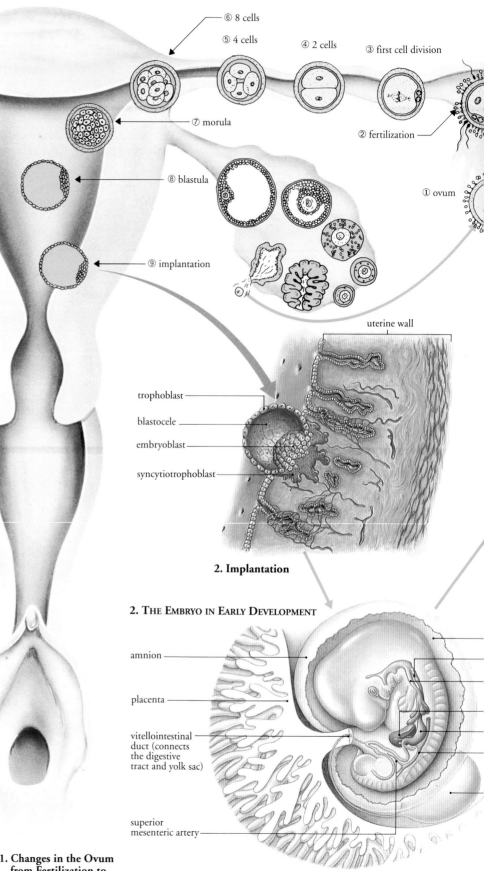

1. FROM FERTILIZATION TO IMPLANTATION

- ⑥ 8 cells
- ⑤ 4 cells
- ④ 2 cells
- ③ first cell division
- ⑦ morula
- ② fertilization
- ① ovum
- ⑧ blastula
- ⑨ implantation

uterine wall

- trophoblast
- blastocele
- embryoblast
- syncytiotrophoblast

2. Implantation

2. THE EMBRYO IN EARLY DEVELOPMENT

- amnion
- placenta
- vitellointestinal duct (connects the digestive tract and yolk sac)
- superior mesenteric artery

From the second week through the eighth week the fertilized ovum is called an embryo. From the ninth week it is known as a fetus. The major organs of the body are almost all formed in the embryotic stage.

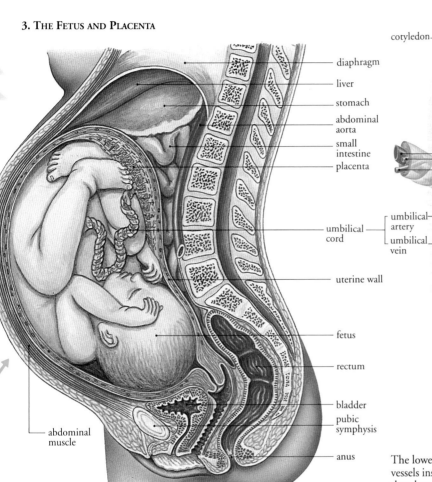

3. THE FETUS AND PLACENTA

- diaphragm
- liver
- stomach
- abdominal aorta
- small intestine
- placenta
- umbilical cord { umbilical artery / umbilical vein }
- uterine wall
- fetus
- rectum
- bladder
- pubic symphysis
- anus
- abdominal muscle

— amnion
— chorionic plate
— uterine artery (spiral artery)
— basal decidua
— myometrium
— uterine vein
— placental septa
— intervillous spaces
— anchoring villus
— villous stem
— free villus

- cotyledon

— amniotic cavity
— esophagus
— trachea
— liver
— stomach
— abdominal aorta
— yolk sac

The lower part of the figure shows the blood vessels inside a cotyledon. In the fetus, blood that has lost oxygen (venous blood) flows through the arteries, whereas blood rich in oxygen and nutrients (arterial blood) flows through the veins. Thus the arteries are shown in blue and the veins are shown in red.

5. CIRCULATION OF BLOOD IN THE PLACENTA

Fetal blood circulates in the blood vessels in the villi of the placenta, and maternal blood fills only the intervillous spaces of the placenta, so there is no direct contact between the two circulations. Exchange of gas and other materials occurs through three cell layers, the endothelium of the fetal blood vessels, intervillous matter, and villous epithelium. Red arrows indicate the flow of arterial blood and blue arrows indicate the flow of venous blood.

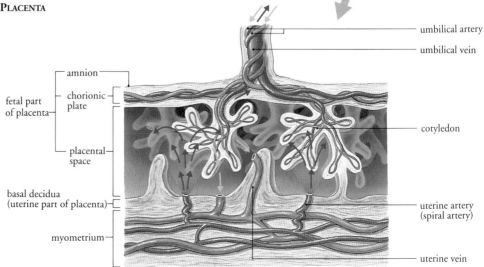

- fetal part of placenta { amnion / chorionic plate / placental space }
- basal decidua (uterine part of placenta)
- myometrium

— umbilical artery
— umbilical vein
— cotyledon
— uterine artery (spiral artery)
— uterine vein

4 The Upper and Lower Limbs

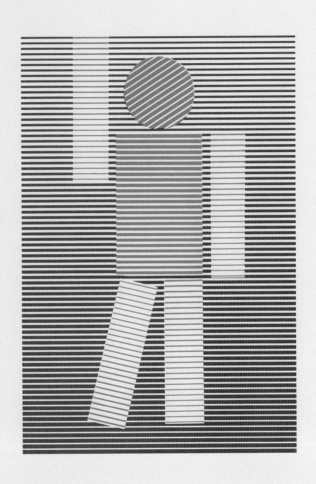

The Bones and Muscles of the Upper and Lower Limbs

1. MAJOR BONES AND MUSCLES OF THE UPPER LIMBS

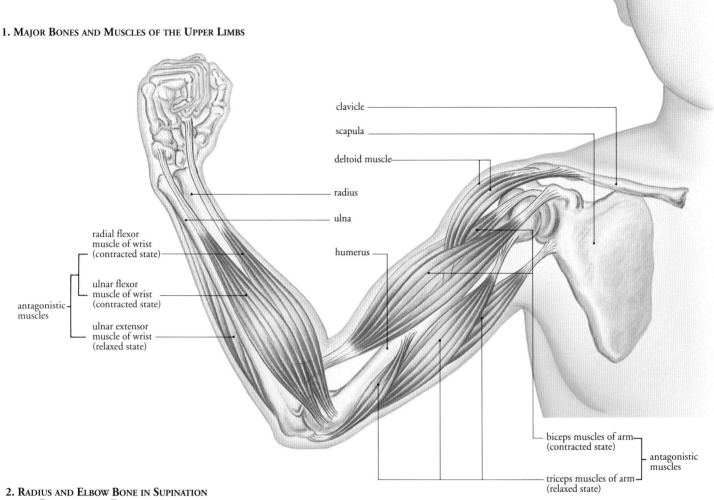

clavicle

scapula

deltoid muscle

radius

ulna

humerus

radial flexor muscle of wrist (contracted state)

ulnar flexor muscle of wrist (contracted state)

ulnar extensor muscle of wrist (relaxed state)

antagonistic muscles

biceps muscles of arm (contracted state)

triceps muscles of arm (relaxed state)

antagonistic muscles

2. RADIUS AND ELBOW BONE IN SUPINATION AND PRONATION OF FOREARM

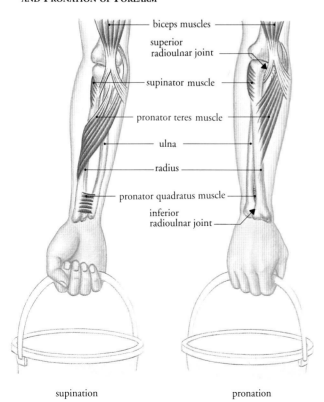

biceps muscles

superior radioulnar joint

supinator muscle

pronator teres muscle

ulna

radius

pronator quadratus muscle

inferior radioulnar joint

supination

pronation

Supination occurs as a result of contraction of the biceps and supinator muscles, and pronation is the result of contraction of the pronator teres and pronator quadratus muscles. These movements center around the radioulnar joints of the elbow. In supination and pronation, the radius and ulna work together in a twisting motion.

The upper limbs consist of pairs of upper arms, forearms, and hands; whereas the lower limbs comprise pairs of thighs, calves, and feet. The operation of the groups of muscles that move the arm bones allows the skillful use of the hands. The lower limbs provide support and mobility for the body.

MAJOR BONES OF THE UPPER LIMBS

Three major bones are in each upper limb: the humerus, ulna, and radius. The large head of the humerus fits in the joint cavity of the scapula at the shoulder and is connected to the ulna and radius at the elbow. The ulna and radius form a joint at the wrist, carpus, which is a collection of eight small bones. The carpus is connected to the metacarpus and the bones of the fingers.

MAJOR MUSCLES OF THE UPPER LIMBS

DELTOID MUSCLE. The deltoid muscle surrounds the lateral, anterior, and posterior sides of the shoulder joint, forming a triangle with its base at the shoulder and its tip facing in the direction of the hand. It functions mainly during abduction (outward lifting) and circumduction (rotational movement toward the front or rear).

TRICEPS AND BICEPS OF THE ARM. The triceps muscles are

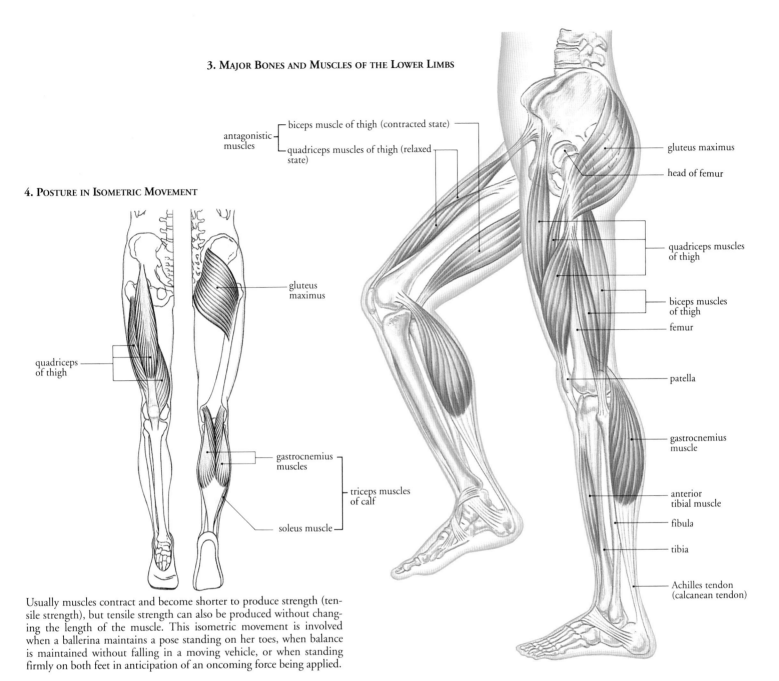

antagonistic muscles
- biceps muscle of thigh (contracted state)
- quadriceps muscles of thigh (relaxed state)

4. POSTURE IN ISOMETRIC MOVEMENT

gluteus maximus

quadriceps of thigh

gastrocnemius muscles

soleus muscle

triceps muscles of calf

gluteus maximus

head of femur

quadriceps muscles of thigh

biceps muscles of thigh

femur

patella

gastrocnemius muscle

anterior tibial muscle

fibula

tibia

Achilles tendon (calcanean tendon)

Usually muscles contract and become shorter to produce strength (tensile strength), but tensile strength can also be produced without changing the length of the muscle. This isometric movement is involved when a ballerina maintains a pose standing on her toes, when balance is maintained without falling in a moving vehicle, or when standing firmly on both feet in anticipation of an oncoming force being applied.

at the back of the upper arm when the arm is held close to the body with the palm of the hand facing front. The large muscles at the front of the upper arm that protrude upward when the elbow is flexed are the biceps. These two sets of muscles work antagonistically, i.e., when the biceps contract, the triceps relax, flexing the elbow joint; when the triceps contract, the biceps relax, extending the elbow joint.

PRONATOR AND SUPINATOR MUSCLES. When a person is standing with arms at the sides and turns the palm toward the rear (pronation), the motion is governed by the pronator teres and the pronator quadratus muscles; supination (the opposite of pronation) is controlled by the supinator muscle and the biceps.

MAJOR BONES OF THE LOWER LIMBS

The major bones of each lower limb include the femur, tibia, and fibula as well as bones of the foot. The femur is the largest bone in the human body. The top of the head of the femur turns an angle of 160°, and the tip becomes part of the hip joint. The distal end is connected to the calf at the knee joint.

The thick tibia and thin fibula comprise the bones of the calf. The former tibia provides almost all the support. The distal end

(lateral malleolus) of the fibula is attached to the tibia with connective tissue so it cannot move.

MAJOR MUSCLES OF THE LOWER LIMBS

GLUTEUS MAXIMUS. The gluteus maximus is the strong thick muscle located on the dorsal side of the buttocks. It moves the hip joint as well as the knee joint and is a major factor in enabling humans to walk upright.

QUADRICEPS AND BICEPS MUSCLES OF THIGH. The quadriceps muscles are located on the front of the thigh and the biceps are located in the rear. These long muscles are antagonistic muscles that govern extension and flexion of the knee joint.

GASTROCNEMIUS MUSCLES, SOLEUS MUSCLE. These muscles are found on the posterior side of the lower leg (calf); the soleus muscle lies deep, whereas the gastrocnemius muscles are closer to the surface. Together these muscles are called the triceps muscles of the calf. At the distal end these muscles become the Achilles tendon (calcaneal tendon), which is attached to the heel bone. These muscles work together to flex the foot.

Major Disorders: contracture of deltoid muscle, contracture of quadriceps muscle of thigh, contracture of gluteus.

The Shoulder Joint

1. STRUCTURE OF THE SHOULDER JOINT

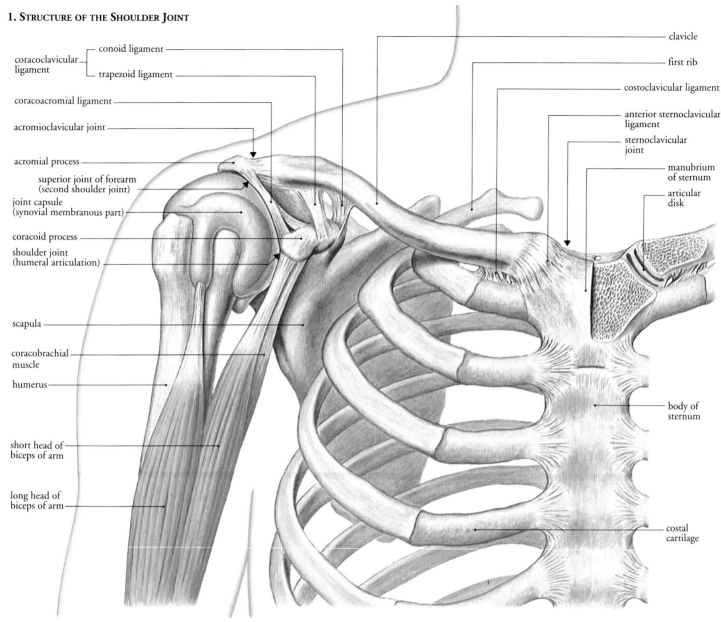

coracoclavicular ligament
— conoid ligament
— trapezoid ligament

coracoacromial ligament

acromioclavicular joint

acromial process

superior joint of forearm
(second shoulder joint)

joint capsule
(synovial membranous part)

coracoid process

shoulder joint
(humeral articulation)

scapula

coracobrachial muscle

humerus

short head of biceps of arm

long head of biceps of arm

clavicle

first rib

costoclavicular ligament

anterior sternoclavicular ligament

sternoclavicular joint

manubrium of sternum

articular disk

body of sternum

costal cartilage

In anatomical terms the shoulder joint indicates the articulation of the head of the humerus and the glenoid cavity of the scapula, but when most people speak of the shoulder joint they also mean the ligaments, tendons, and bones that make up the pectoral girdle, such as the acromioclavicular joint, the superior joint of the forearm, and the sternoclavicular joint, all of which participate in giving rise to a wide variety of movement.

2. SHOULDER JOINT AND VICINITY VIEWED FROM ABOVE

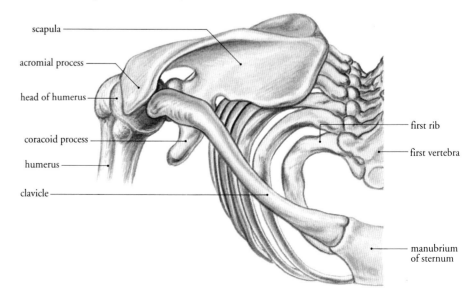

scapula

acromial process

head of humerus

coracoid process

humerus

clavicle

first rib

first vertebra

manubrium of sternum

3. STRUCTURE OF THE SCAPULA

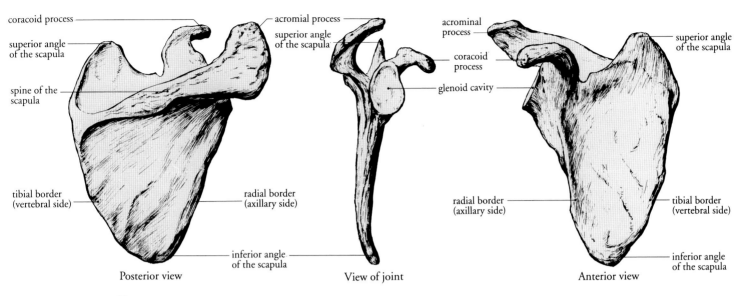

coracoid process

superior angle
of the scapula

spine of the
scapula

tibial border
(vertebral side)

radial border
(axillary side)

inferior angle
of the scapula

Posterior view

acromial process

superior angle
of the scapula

View of joint

glenoid cavity

acrominal
process

coracoid
process

radial border
(axillary side)

Anterior view

superior angle
of the scapula

tibial border
(vertebral side)

inferior angle
of the scapula

4. MOVEMENT OF THE HUMERUS AND CLAVICLE WHEN RAISING THE ARM

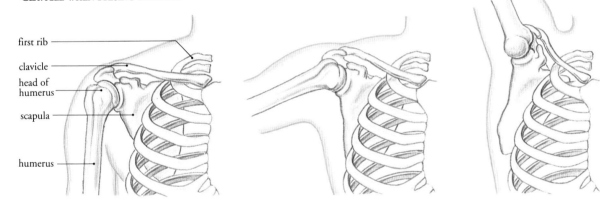

first rib

clavicle

head of
humerus

scapula

humerus

The shoulder joint is capable of the widest range of movement of any joint in the body. The scapula and clavicle are responsible for the range of movement. In particular, when raising the arm from a horizontal position the bones interlock, allowing the arm to be raised straight up.

As humans began to walk in the upright position the roles of the upper and lower limbs diverged to allow unrestricted use of the hands. The shoulder joint makes this possible.

Structure. The large, almost perfectly round head of the humerus and the relatively small and shallow glenoid cavity that lies on the lateral side of the scapula make up the shoulder joint. The acromial process and coracoid process project out from the scapula like eaves over the shoulder joint, and together with the glenoidal labrium the ligaments (bands of tissue that fortify the joints) like the one connecting these two processes help make up for the relatively small size of the glenoid cavity.

Function. In the working position of the upper limbs, the center of the glenoid cavity is not on the frontal plane but directly oblique fore and lateral. It is much easier to move the shoulder joint around the axis that passes through the center of the humerus head and the center of the glenoid cavity. This position is known as the "working position" of the upper limbs. When one writes or holds a fork the humerus automatically assumes this position.

Range of Movement. The shoulder joint is a ball-and-socket joint in which the round head of the humerus fits into the socket of the glenoid of the scapula. Although it may appear as though movement is possible in all directions, it is restricted by support-

ing structures such as the coracoacromial ligaments located near the joint (e.g., the arm can be raised vertically in the posterior direction only as high as a 50° angle). Movement of the shoulder joint alone allows the arm to be raised in the lateral direction only as far as 90°, but the acromioclavicular joint and the sternoclavicular joint work together to allow the arm to be raised to 180°. In this way, movement of the upper arm is the result not just of the shoulder joint itself, but also of cooperation between the sternoclavicular and acromioclavicular joints and the superior joint of the forearm (formed by the coracoid process and the head of the humerus) as well as the sliding of the humerus at the posterior side of the thorax (Figure 4).

Dislocation of the Shoulder Joint. Muscles involved in the movement of the shoulder joint are found on the lateral side of the joint; these muscles also stabilize the joint. They are well developed on the upper and posterior sides of the shoulder, but they are weak on the ventral and lower sides. A strong outside force can cause the head of the humerus to slip out of the glenoid cavity. This is known as dislocation.

Major Disorders: frozen shoulder, cervicobrachial syndrome, rotator cuff injury, baseball shoulder, supraspinatus syndrome, Sprengel's deformity.

The Elbow Joint and Joint of the Hand

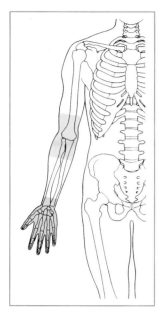

1. STRUCTURE OF THE ELBOW JOINT (RIGHT ELBOW)

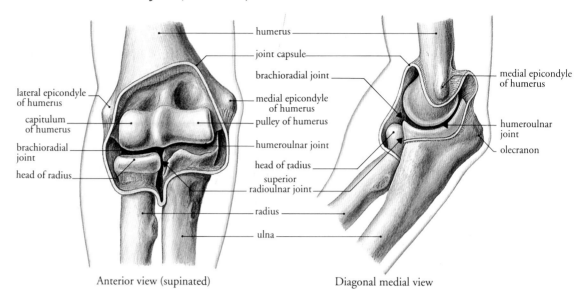

humerus

joint capsule

brachioradial joint

medial epicondyle of humerus

pulley of humerus

humeroulnar joint

head of radius

superior radioulnar joint

radius

ulna

lateral epicondyle of humerus

capitulum of humerus

brachioradial joint

head of radius

Anterior view (supinated)

medial epicondyle of humerus

humeroulnar joint

olecranon

Diagonal medial view

2. LIGAMENTS OF THE ELBOW JOINT (RIGHT ELBOW)

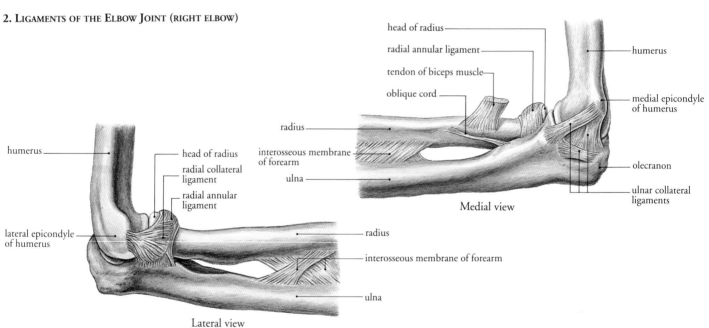

humerus

head of radius

radial collateral ligament

radial annular ligament

lateral epicondyle of humerus

radius

interosseous membrane of forearm

ulna

Lateral view

head of radius

radial annular ligament

tendon of biceps muscle

oblique cord

radius

interosseous membrane of forearm

ulna

humerus

medial epicondyle of humerus

olecranon

ulnar collateral ligaments

Medial view

ELBOW JOINT

The elbow joint is the juncture between the upper arm and the forearm, and it functions to move the forearm.

Structure. The elbow joint, a compound joint, is the articulation of three bones, the humerus, the radius, and the ulna. The joint is covered by a common joint capsule. The axis of the distal end (toward the hand) of the humerus is inclined forward at an angle of approx 45° in relation to the longitudinal axis of the bone. As a result it is easier to flex than to extend.

Function. Flexing and extending the elbow is done by the decranal joint, which connects the humerus and the ulna. It operates like a single-axis hinge. The radioulnar joint formed by the radius and the ulna is responsible for supination (rotating the palm of the hand toward the front) and pronation (rotating the palm toward the rear). This radioulnar joint is a pivot joint, which means it allows

rotary motion on one plane only. The axis of this supination and pronation does not pass through the center of the humerus but through the line connecting the proximal end (toward the shoulder) of the radius and the distal end of the ulna. The range of movement of the elbow joint is narrow compared with that of the shoulder joint. When the elbow is flexed and the hand is brought up, the arm can bend about 145°. In the opposite direction, however, the forearm can be extended only about 5°. Furthermore, supination and pronation are limited to a range of 90°. The elbow joint plays an important part in our daily lives, making it possible for us to perform a variety of physical acts. For example, when using a cane, the elbow is extended, and when washing a car, it is flexed; writing calls for pronation, whereas holding a bowl of food requires supination.

Major Disorders: pulled elbow, cubitus varus, cubitus valgus, baseball elbow, tennis elbow.

3. Bones and Joints of the Right Hand

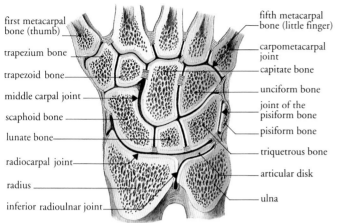

first metacarpal bone (thumb)
trapezium bone
trapezoid bone
middle carpal joint
scaphoid bone
lunate bone
radiocarpal joint
radius
inferior radioulnar joint

fifth metacarpal bone (little finger)
carpometacarpal joint
capitate bone
unciform bone
joint of the pisiform bone
pisiform bone
triquetrous bone
articular disk
ulna

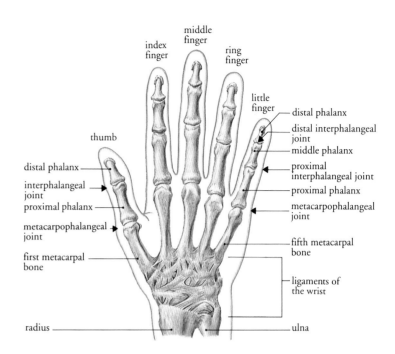

index finger
middle finger
ring finger
little finger
thumb
distal phalanx
interphalangeal joint
proximal phalanx
metacarpophalangeal joint
first metacarpal bone
radius

distal phalanx
distal interphalangeal joint
middle phalanx
proximal interphalangeal joint
proximal phalanx
metacarpophalangeal joint
fifth metacarpal bone
ligaments of the wrist
ulna

The figure above is a horizontal sectional view of the back of the hand, and the figure to the right shows a posterior view of the bones and the ligaments of the carpus. The distal phalanges, middle phalanges, and proximal phalanges together comprise the bones of the fingers. The thumb, however, unlike the other four fingers, does not have a middle phalanx and one of the interphalangeal joints.

4. Tendon Sheaths of the Hand

In the back of the hand as well as in the palm are sheaths containing tendons (tendon sheaths). The synovial fluid within these sheaths allows the flexor and extensor tendons (which extend and flex the fingers) and abductor muscles to move smoothly. If the tendon sheath becomes inflamed, the fine movements of the hand may be limited. The extensor retinaculum, flexor retinaculum, and pars annularis vaginae fibrosae prevent the tendons from rising during flexion and extension.

1. Tendon Sheaths of the Back of the Hand

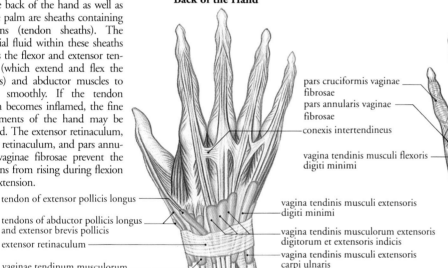

pars cruciformis vaginae fibrosae
pars annularis vaginae fibrosae
conexis intertendineus
vagina tendinis musculi flexoris digiti minimi
vagina tendinis musculi extensoris digiti minimi
vagina tendinis musculorum extensoris digitorum et extensoris indicis
vagina tendinis musculi extensoris carpi ulnaris

tendon of extensor pollicis longus
tendons of abductor pollicis longus and extensor brevis pollicis
extensor retinaculum
vaginae tendinum musculorum extensoris carpi radialium

2. Tendon Sheaths of the Palm of the Hand

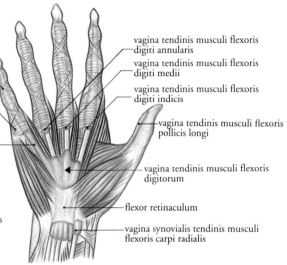

vagina tendinis musculi flexoris digiti annularis
vagina tendinis musculi flexoris digiti medii
vagina tendinis musculi flexoris digiti indicis
vagina tendinis musculi flexoris pollicis longi
vagina tendinis musculi flexoris digitorum
flexor retinaculum
vagina synovialis tendinis musculi flexoris carpi radialis

Joints of the Hand

The human hand is uniquely capable of exceptionally fine movements. The wrists have joints for flexing, extending, and rotary movement, and the fingers have smaller joints for flexing and extending in a variety of positions.

Structure. The joints of the hand include the joints formed by the radius of the forearm and the eight carpal bones of the wrist. Generally, when we speak of the joints of the hand we mean the radiocarpal joint formed by the radius and three carpal bones (the scaphoid, lunate, and triquetal bones) plus the S-shaped middle carpal joint that runs between the carpal bone close to the fingers and the carpal bone close to the radius.

JOINTS OF THE FINGERS. The joints of the fingers are between the distal, middle, and proximal phalanges and between the metacarpal bones and the carpal bones. These joints make possible the subtle movements of the fingers. The movement of the thumb distinguishes humans from the rest of the animal world.

This movement is the function of the carpometacarpal joint, located between the metacarpal bone of the thumb and the trapezium bone (one of the carpal bones).

Function. The most important functions of the hand are obtaining sensory information by touch and grasping objects. The palm of the hand is used mainly for feeling and gripping. The hand can also be used to communicate feelings and thoughts.

The joints of the hand allow the wrist to extend, adduct, and abduct. The carpometacarpal joint of the thumb allows it to flex and extend as well as adduct (bring the thumb close to the index finger) and abduct (move the thumb at a right angle with the palm). The wide range of movements that the hand is capable of greatly increase its usefulness. Synovial fluid contained in the tendon sheaths of the hand enable these movements to be performed smoothly.

Major Disorders: rheumatism, Dupuytren's contracture, tendovaginitis, trigger finger, Kienböck's disease.

The Hip Joint and Knee Joint

1. STRUCTURE OF THE HIP JOINT

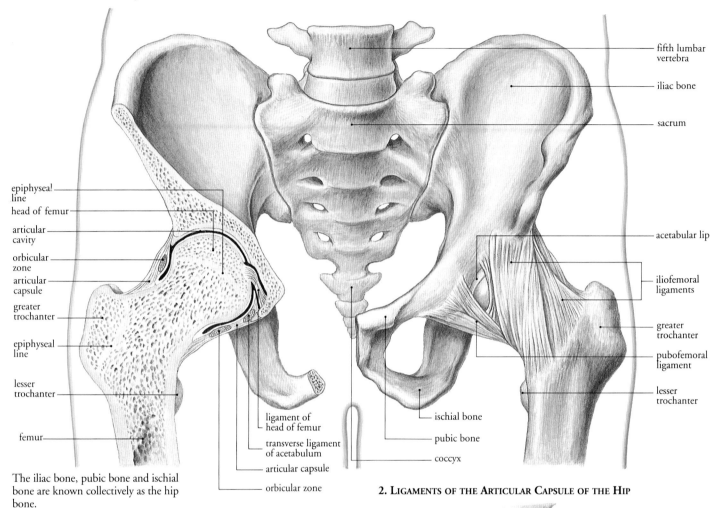

fifth lumbar vertebra

iliac bone

sacrum

acetabular lip

iliofemoral ligaments

greater trochanter

pubofemoral ligament

lesser trochanter

epiphyseal line

head of femur

articular cavity

orbicular zone

articular capsule

greater trochanter

epiphyseal line

lesser trochanter

femur

ligament of head of femur

transverse ligament of acetabulum

articular capsule

orbicular zone

ischial bone

pubic bone

coccyx

The iliac bone, pubic bone and ischial bone are known collectively as the hip bone.

2. LIGAMENTS OF THE ARTICULAR CAPSULE OF THE HIP

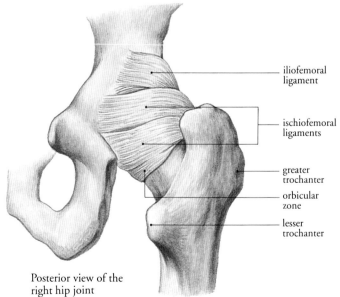

iliofemoral ligament

ischiofemoral ligaments

greater trochanter

orbicular zone

lesser trochanter

Posterior view of the right hip joint

HIP JOINT

The hip joint joins the lower limbs to the body and performs the important function of making it possible for humans to walk on two legs.

Structure. The hip joint is formed by the acetabulum (cotyloid cavity) of the pelvis and the head of the femur. The acetabulum opens at approx a 42° angle from the horizontal plane in the lateral, inferior, and ventral directions. The head of the femur (articular head) fits inside this cavity to form the joint. Like the shoulder joint, the hip joint is a ball-and-socket joint. The acetabulum is deep, and approximately two-thirds of the bone's head fits inside. Three strong ligaments attached to the lateral side of the joint capsule stabilize the joint, and the capsule broadly envelopes the head of the femur. In contrast, the shoulder joint has a shallow glenoid cavity and is easy to dislocate. The distribution of blood vessels is limited in the narrow section between the bone head and trochanter, which is one reason why fracture of the neck of the femur occurs more easily among the elderly.

Function. Although the risk of dislocation of the hip is limited because the head of the joint is situated deep within the cavity, the added stability limits the joint's range of movement despite the fact that it is a ball-and-socket joint. Since human beings began placing the weight of the entire body on the lower limbs and walking on two legs, the evolutionary process pro-gressed in favor of durability over refined movement. When the knee joint is flexed the range of movement of the hip joint is roughly double that when the knee joint is extended because the tension of the powerful muscles of the thigh is diminished.

Major Disorders: aseptic or avascular necrosis of the femoral head, congenital dislocation of hip, Perthes' disease, aplasia of acetabulum, coxa valga, coxa vara, osteoarthritis.

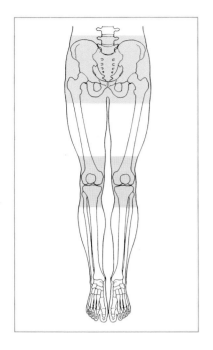

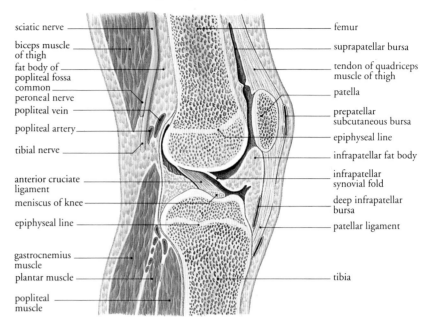

sciatic nerve

biceps muscle of thigh

fat body of popliteal fossa

common peroneal nerve

popliteal vein

popliteal artery

tibial nerve

anterior cruciate ligament

meniscus of knee

epiphyseal line

gastrocnemius muscle

plantar muscle

popliteal muscle

femur

suprapatellar bursa

tendon of quadriceps muscle of thigh

patella

prepatellar subcutaneous bursa

epiphyseal line

infrapatellar fat body

infrapatellar synovial fold

deep infrapatellar bursa

patellar ligament

tibia

4. Ligaments of Knee Joint (right knee)

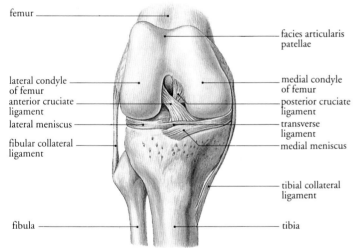

femur

facies articularis patellae

lateral condyle of femur

anterior cruciate ligament

lateral meniscus

fibular collateral ligament

medial condyle of femur

posterior cruciate ligament

transverse ligament

medial meniscus

tibial collateral ligament

fibula

tibia

Anterior view with patella removed

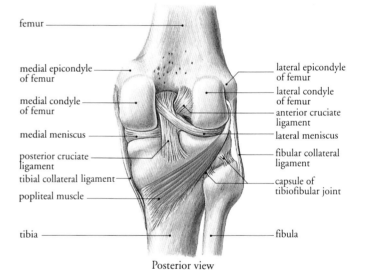

femur

medial epicondyle of femur

medial condyle of femur

medial meniscus

posterior cruciate ligament

tibial collateral ligament

popliteal muscle

tibia

lateral epicondyle of femur

lateral condyle of femur

anterior cruciate ligament

lateral meniscus

fibular collateral ligament

capsule of tibiofibular joint

fibula

Posterior view

KNEE JOINT

Structure. The knee joint connects the femur, which is the longest long bone of the human body, and the tibia, the second longest bone. The patella is located inside the tendon sheath of the quadriceps muscles at the front of the thigh and is also part of the knee structure. When viewed from the front, the medial and lateral condyles of the femur look like two tires standing side by side. When viewed from the side, the knee joint is seen to protrude.

The lateral condyle of the tibia at the knee joint is concave, whereas the medial condyle is convex. These surfaces are not compatible with the surfaces at the end of the femur, resulting in considerable space between the two bones (articular cavity). At the joint, two circular menisci made of fibrous cartilage are attached to the tibia. Membranous folds containing fatty material extend from the joint capsule, and interarticular ligaments (anterior and posterior cruciate ligaments of the knee) stabilize the bones inside the articular cavity.

Function. The knee joint, located between the hip and ankle

joints, is capable of flexion and extension movement that ranges from sitting with the knees folded under to standing upright. The knee is also the joint that bears the most weight in the body. For these reasons, a high degree of stability is required by the knees. The knee joint is most stable when it is completely extended, and it is able to maintain a standing position without the tension of the quadriceps muscles of the thigh.

Outside the joint various ligaments, the patellar ligament in front and the fibular collateral ligament and patellar retinacula at the medial and lateral sides, reinforce the knee and help prevent dislocation.

The patella is the disk-shaped bone of the knee that can be moved slightly with the fingers. It functions to relieve friction between the bones and muscles when the knee is flexed and extended.

Major Disorders: pulled knee, osteochondritis of the knee, rheumatoid arthritis of the knee, chondromalacia, patellae, hydrarthrosis of the knee, congenital dislocation of the knee.

The Foot

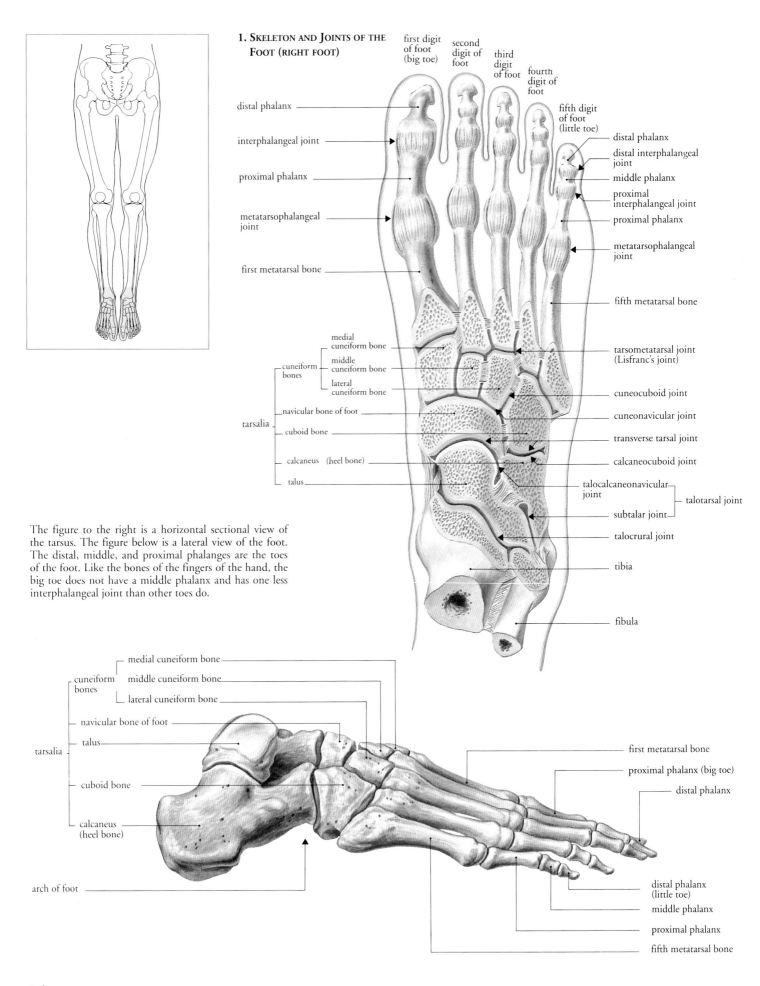

1. SKELETON AND JOINTS OF THE FOOT (RIGHT FOOT)

first digit of foot (big toe)

second digit of foot

third digit of foot

fourth digit of foot

fifth digit of foot (little toe)

distal phalanx

interphalangeal joint

proximal phalanx

metatarsophalangeal joint

first metatarsal bone

distal phalanx

distal interphalangeal joint

middle phalanx

proximal interphalangeal joint

proximal phalanx

metatarsophalangeal joint

fifth metatarsal bone

cuneiform bones
- medial cuneiform bone
- middle cuneiform bone
- lateral cuneiform bone

tarsalia
- navicular bone of foot
- cuboid bone
- calcaneus (heel bone)
- talus

tarsometatarsal joint (Lisfranc's joint)

cuneocuboid joint

cuneonavicular joint

transverse tarsal joint

calcaneocuboid joint

talocalcaneonavicular joint

subtalar joint

talotarsal joint

talocrural joint

tibia

fibula

The figure to the right is a horizontal sectional view of the tarsus. The figure below is a lateral view of the foot. The distal, middle, and proximal phalanges are the toes of the foot. Like the bones of the fingers of the hand, the big toe does not have a middle phalanx and has one less interphalangeal joint than other toes do.

cuneiform bones
- medial cuneiform bone
- middle cuneiform bone
- lateral cuneiform bone

tarsalia
- navicular bone of foot
- talus
- cuboid bone
- calcaneus (heel bone)

arch of foot

first metatarsal bone

proximal phalanx (big toe)

distal phalanx

distal phalanx (little toe)

middle phalanx

proximal phalanx

fifth metatarsal bone

2. Section of Achilles Tendon and Vicinity

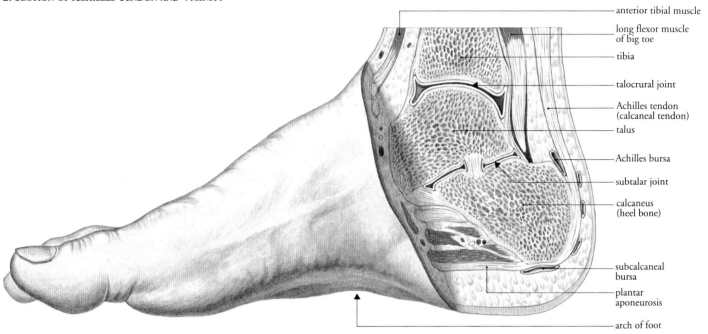

- anterior tibial muscle
- long flexor muscle of big toe
- tibia
- talocrural joint
- Achilles tendon (calcaneal tendon)
- talus
- Achilles bursa
- subtalar joint
- calcaneus (heel bone)
- subcalcaneal bursa
- plantar aponeurosis
- arch of foot

3. Major Ligaments of the Joints of the Foot

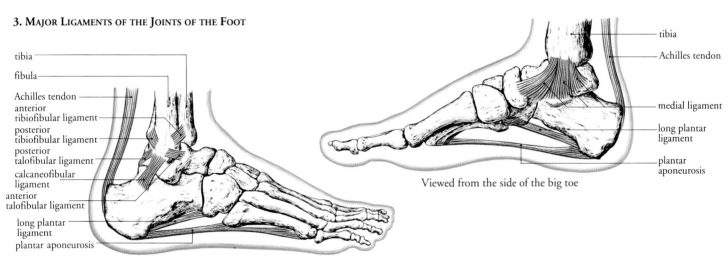

- tibia
- fibula
- Achilles tendon
- anterior ribiofibular ligament
- posterior tibiofibular ligament
- posterior talofibular ligament
- calcaneofibular ligament
- anterior talofibular ligament
- long plantar ligament
- plantar aponeurosis

Viewed from the side of the little toe

- tibia
- Achilles tendon
- medial ligament
- long plantar ligament
- plantar aponeurosis

Viewed from the side of the big toe

JOINTS OF THE FOOT

The joints of the foot are the ankle (connect the lower leg [crus] and the foot) and the joints of the digits of the foot.

Structure. The foot joints are formed by the tibia and fibula of the lower leg and the seven bones of the ankle. The main joints of the foot are the talocrural joint and the talonavicular joint, which are formed by the talus and navicular bones. In addition, the tarsometatarsal joints formed by the various metatarsal and tarsal bones form a strong arch with powerful connecting ligaments. The arch acts as a shock absorber and supports the body on the ground.

JOINTS OF THE TOES. The range of movement of the joints of the toes is not as wide as that of the joints of the fingers, e.g., movement of the big toe is limited. However, they work with the other joints of the foot to enable smooth progress when walking.

Function. Over time, evolution has changed the foot more than any other part of the upper or lower limbs. The human foot and the foot of a few other primates differ considerably from the feet of four-footed animals. The primate foot functions as a plate for maintaining a horizontal position, enabling the longitudinal axis of the lower leg to be held in a near perpendicular position. The tarsal and metatarsal bones protrude to form a long narrow vault on the back of the foot surrounded by tarsophalangeal extensor tendons, blood vessels, and lymphatic vessels. The arch of the sole of the foot allows it to resist the great pressure put on it by the weight of the body. Along its length and breadth the arch is supported by ligaments, tendons, and muscles. At birth, the arch is usually flat but it develops with age. The foot also has numerous muscles for moving the toes, and characteristic proper muscles are found at both the median and lateral edges.

The talocrural joint of the foot is a hinge joint with a transverse axis and works to flex and extend the foot. The talonavicular joint moves on an axis that lies diagonally to the longitudinal axis of the foot and can invert and evert the foot.

Major Disorders: congenital foot deformities such as clubfoot (talipes valgus, talipes varus), flat foot, gout, plantar aponeurositis.

The Blood Vessels of the Upper Limbs

**1. BIFURCATIONS AND ROUTES OF THE
ARTERIES AND VEINS OF THE UPPER LIMBS**

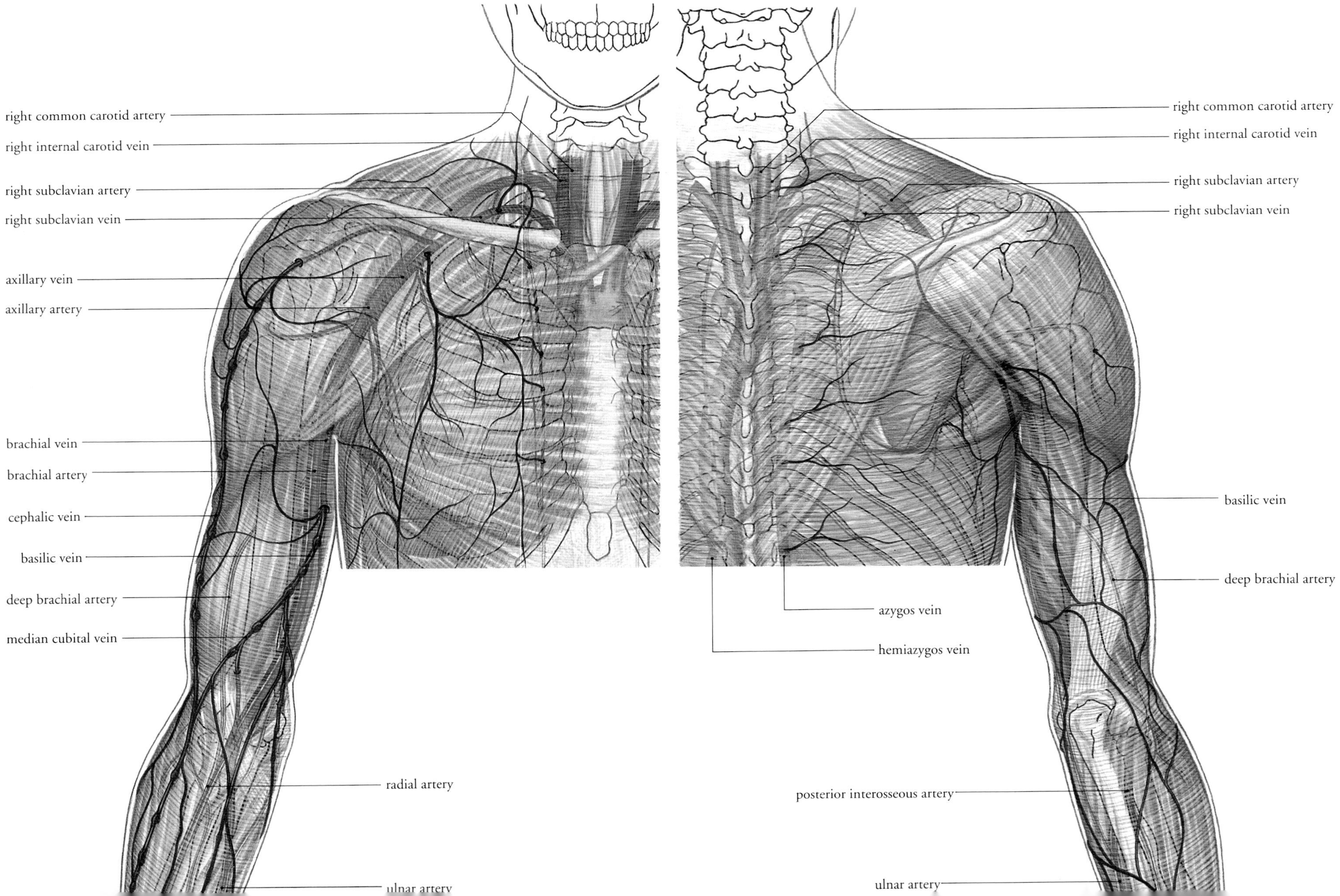

right common carotid artery

right internal carotid vein

right subclavian artery

right subclavian vein

basilic vein

deep brachial artery

azygos vein

hemiazygos vein

posterior interosseous artery

ulnar artery

right common carotid artery

right internal carotid vein

right subclavian artery

right subclavian vein

axillary vein

axillary artery

brachial vein

brachial artery

cephalic vein

basilic vein

deep brachial artery

median cubital vein

radial artery

ulnar artery

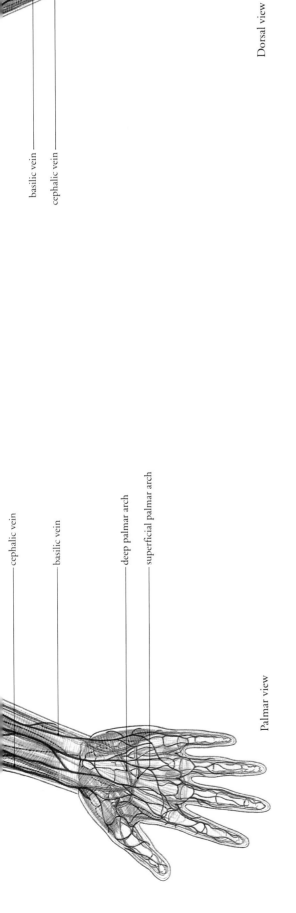

basilic vein

cephalic vein

Dorsal view

cephalic vein

basilic vein

deep palmar arch

superficial palmar arch

Palmar view

Arteries. The name of a single artery changes depending on its location. Branching from the aortic arch, the left subclavian artery is the origin of the arteries of the left upper limb. As it passes under the arm, its name changes to the axillary artery; its name changes again as it passes through the arm, becoming the brachial artery. The brachial artery, protected on the lateral side by the humerus goes as far as the elbow where it divides into the ulnar artery and the radial artery. The ulnar artery further bifurcates into interosseous arteries. These arteries connect with each other (anastomose) in the palm of the hand and form the superficial and deep palmar arches. Thin arteries form arterial networks at various joint regions, including the acromion, elbow joint, and hand joints.

Veins. A venous network collects venous blood from the palm and fingers, becoming the basilic vein. The basilic vein ascends and joins the brachial vein, which joins with the cephalic vein into the axillary vein, and becomes the subclavian vein. The median cubital vein is the vein that diagonally connects the basilic and cephalic veins (which lie close to the surface of the arm). The routes and thickness of these veins differ considerably among individuals.

The Veins Used for Injections. The median cubital vein is often used to give injections because it is easy to see when the upper arm is tied; in addition, it lies in a direction that makes it easy to inject with a hypodermic needle. The basilic and cephalic veins are also used at times. In about 2% of the population the radial artery lies close to the surface, and medication that is supposed to be injected into the vein is injected into the artery by mistake.

2. ARTERIES OF THE DEEP REGION OF THE HAND

proper palmar digital arteries

common palmar digital artery

superficial palmar arch

deep palmar arch

median nerve

ulnar artery

radial artery

ulna

radius

Right hand viewed from the palmar side

3. VEINS OF THE SUPERFICIAL REGION OF THE HAND

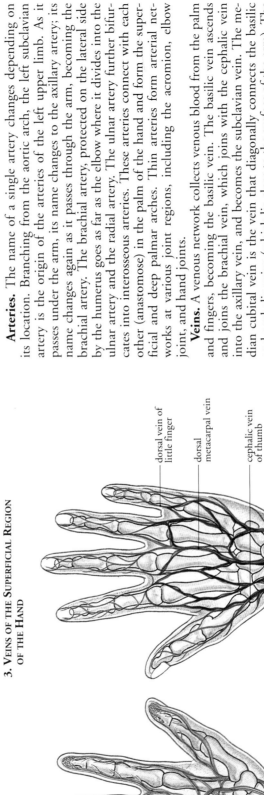

dorsal vein of little finger

dorsal metacarpal vein

cephalic vein of thumb

ulna

radius

Right hand viewed from the opisthenar side

99

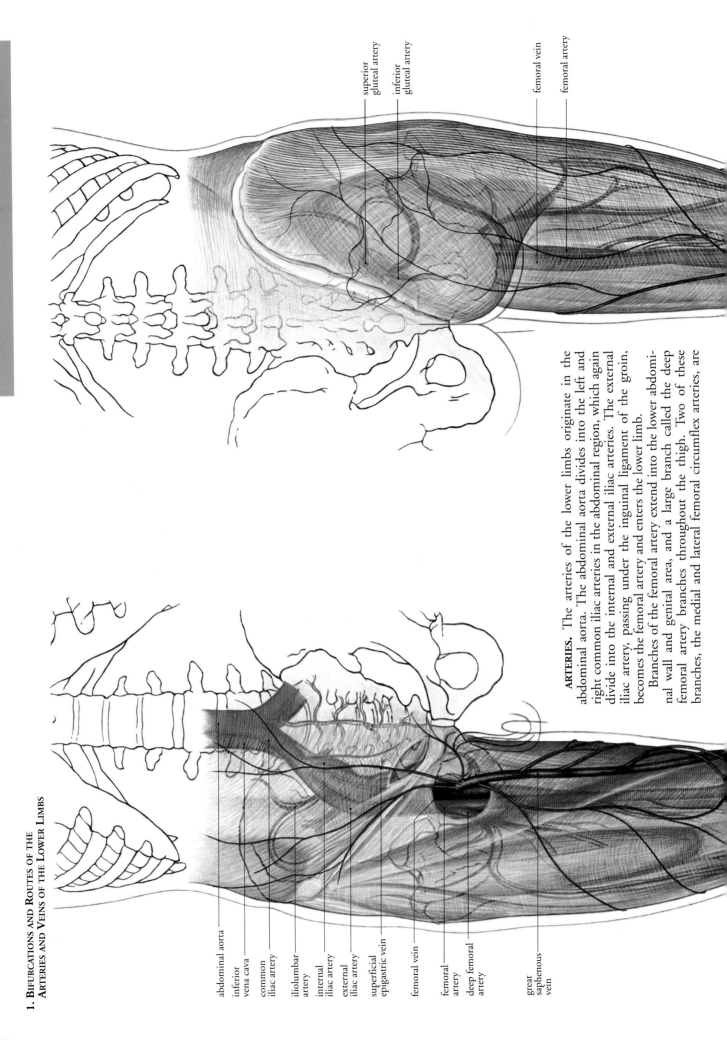

The Blood Vessels of the Lower Limbs

1. BIFURCATIONS AND ROUTES OF THE ARTERIES AND VEINS OF THE LOWER LIMBS

superior gluteal artery

inferior gluteal artery

femoral vein

femoral artery

abdominal aorta

inferior vena cava

common iliac artery

iliolumbar artery

internal iliac artery

external iliac artery

superficial epigastric vein

femoral vein

femoral artery

deep femoral artery

great saphenous vein

ARTERIES. The arteries of the lower limbs originate in the abdominal aorta. The abdominal aorta divides into the left and right common iliac arteries in the abdominal region, which again divide into the internal and external iliac arteries. The external iliac artery, passing under the inguinal ligament of the groin, becomes the femoral artery and enters the lower limb.

Branches of the femoral artery extend into the lower abdominal wall and genital area, and a large branch called the deep femoral artery branches throughout the thigh. Two of these branches, the medial and lateral femoral circumflex arteries, are

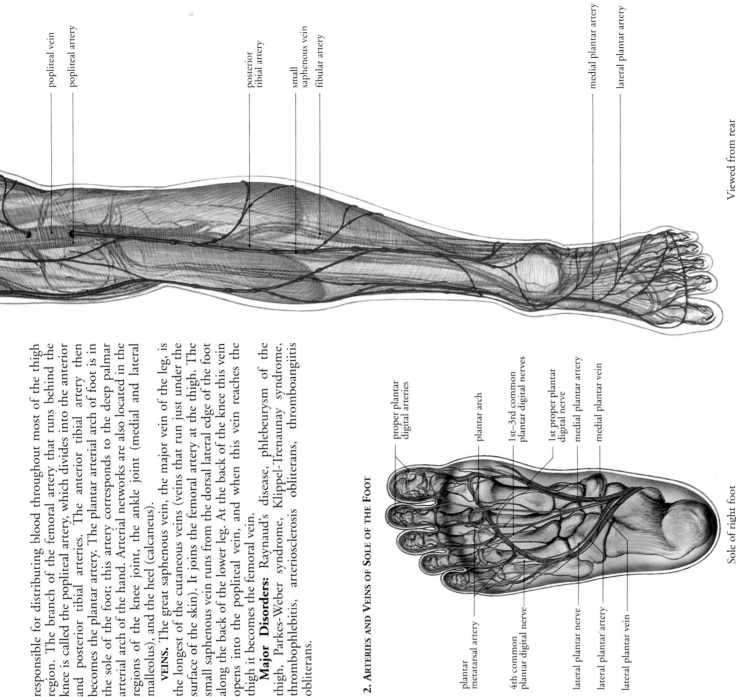

popliteal vein
popliteal artery

posterior tibial artery

small saphenous vein
fibular artery

medial plantar artery
lateral plantar artery

Viewed from rear

descending artery of knee
lateral inferior vein of knee
medial superior artery of knee
lateral inferior vein of knee
medial inferior artery of knee

anterior tibial artery
posterior tibial artery
anterior tibial vein

dorsal artery of foot

dorsal venous arch of foot

Viewed from front

responsible for distributing blood throughout most of the thigh region. The branch of the femoral artery that runs behind the knee is called the popliteal artery, which divides into the anterior and posterior tibial arteries. The anterior tibial artery then becomes the plantar artery. The plantar arterial arch of foot is in the sole of the foot; this artery corresponds to the deep palmar arterial arch of the hand. Arterial networks are also located in the regions of the knee joint, the ankle joint (medial and lateral malleolus), and the heel (calcaneus).

VEINS. The great saphenous vein, the major vein of the leg, is the longest of the cutaneous veins (veins that run just under the surface of the skin). It joins the femoral artery at the thigh. The small saphenous vein runs from the dorsal lateral edge of the foot along the back of the lower leg. At the back of the knee this vein opens into the popliteal vein, and when this vein reaches the thigh it becomes the femoral vein.

Major Disorders: Raynaud's disease, phlebeurysm of the thigh, Parkes-Weber syndrome, Klippel-Trenaunay syndrome, thrombophlebitis, arteriosclerosis obliterans, thromboangiitis obliterans.

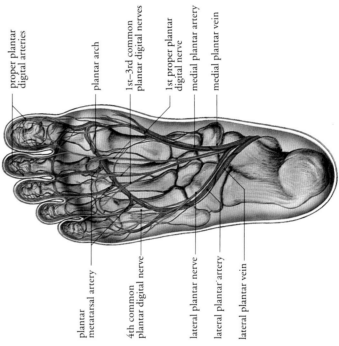

proper plantar digital arteries

plantar arch

1st–3rd common plantar digital nerves

1st proper plantar digital nerve

medial plantar artery

medial plantar vein

plantar metatarsal artery

4th common plantar digital nerve

lateral plantar nerve
lateral plantar artery
lateral plantar vein

Sole of right foot

2. ARTERIES AND VEINS OF SOLE OF THE FOOT

1. BIFURCATIONS AND ROUTES OF THE NERVES OF THE UPPER LIMBS

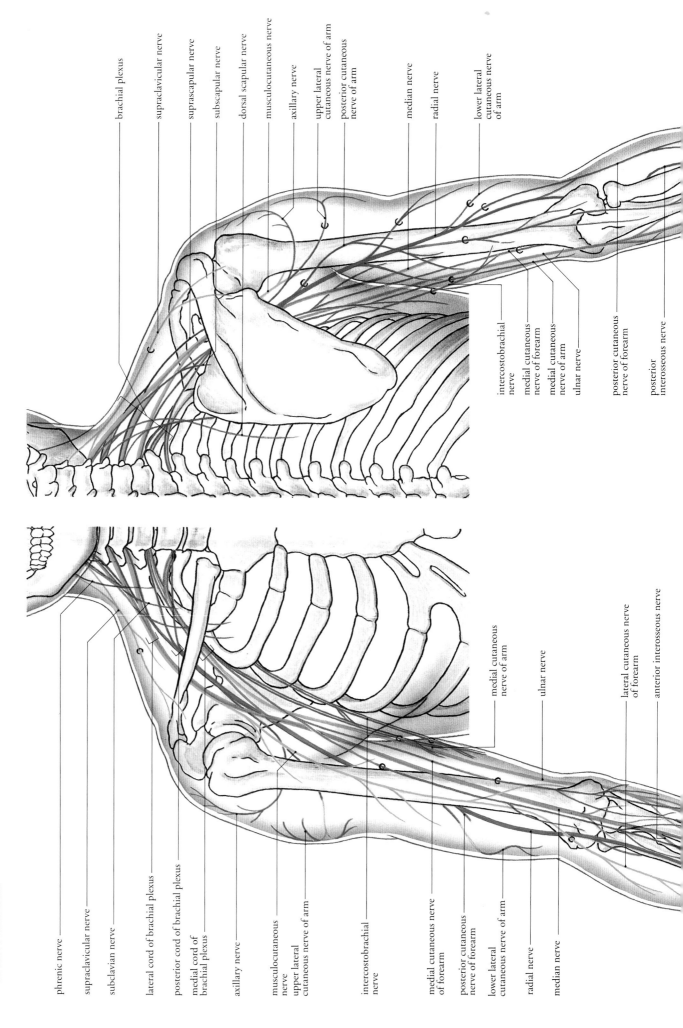

brachial plexus

supraclavicular nerve

suprascapular nerve

subscapular nerve

dorsal scapular nerve

musculocutaneous nerve

axillary nerve

upper lateral cutaneous nerve of arm

posterior cutaneous nerve of arm

median nerve

radial nerve

lower lateral cutaneous nerve of arm

intercostobrachial nerve

medial cutaneous nerve of forearm

medial cutaneous nerve of arm

ulnar nerve

posterior cutaneous nerve of forearm

posterior interosseous nerve

medial cutaneous nerve of arm

ulnar nerve

lateral cutaneous nerve of forearm

anterior interosseous nerve

phrenic nerve

supraclavicular nerve

subclavian nerve

lateral cord of brachial plexus

posterior cord of brachial plexus

medial cord of brachial plexus

axillary nerve

musculocutaneous nerve

upper lateral cutaneous nerve of arm

intercostobrachial nerve

medial cutaneous nerve of forearm

posterior cutaneous nerve of forearm

lower lateral cutaneous nerve of arm

radial nerve

median nerve

dorsal digital nerve

Dorsal view

common palmar digital nerve

proper palmar digital nerve

Palmar view

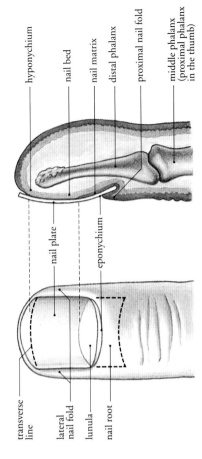

2. STRUCTURE OF THE NAIL

hyponychium

nail bed

nail matrix

distal phalanx

proximal nail fold

middle phalanx (proximal phalanx in the thumb)

nail plate

eponychium

transverse line

lateral nail fold

lunula

nail root

The nail is the general name for the highly differentiated type of skin comprising the nail plate and surrounding tissue. The nail protects the tip of the finger and plays an important role in the sense of touch. If the nail is lost, the sense of touch in the tip of the finger diminishes. The nail is affixed to the nail bed and grows 0.1–0.14 mm per day. If the matrix tissue is destroyed the nail cannot grow back.

As in the rest of the body, both motor nerves (which send commands to the muscles) and sensory nerves (which sense what is felt by the skin and transmit this information to the central nervous system) are distributed throughout the upper limbs.

The nerves that control the shoulder and upper limbs extend from the brachial plexus at the base of the neck. The brachial plexus is a collection of nerves, some from the cervical vertebrae and some from the thoracic vertebrae. The nerves going to the shoulder and those going to the upper limbs diverge at the brachial plexus. The nerves that go to the upper limbs pass behind the clavicle and divide into three bundles—the median, lateral, and posterior nerve bundles. Each nerve bundle is distributed to different parts of the limbs to perform motor and sensory activities. The major nerves of the upper limbs are the ulnar, radial, axillary, median, and musculocutaneous nerves.

Sometimes when the elbow is hit a sensation like an electric shock going toward the little finger is felt. This occurs when the ulnar nerve, which runs from the back of the elbow joint down along the side of the arm to the little finger, has received a direct blow. If the radial nerve is injured, the hand remains in a hanging position and the fingers cannot move (wrist drop). If the median nerve is injured, the area of the palm close to the thumb loses feeling and the thumb cannot bend (ape hand).

The main nerves of the brachial plexus pass through a narrow passage from the spinal cord through the cervical vertebrae. Injury to this area (e.g., in an automobile accident) can stretch and break apart the nerves.

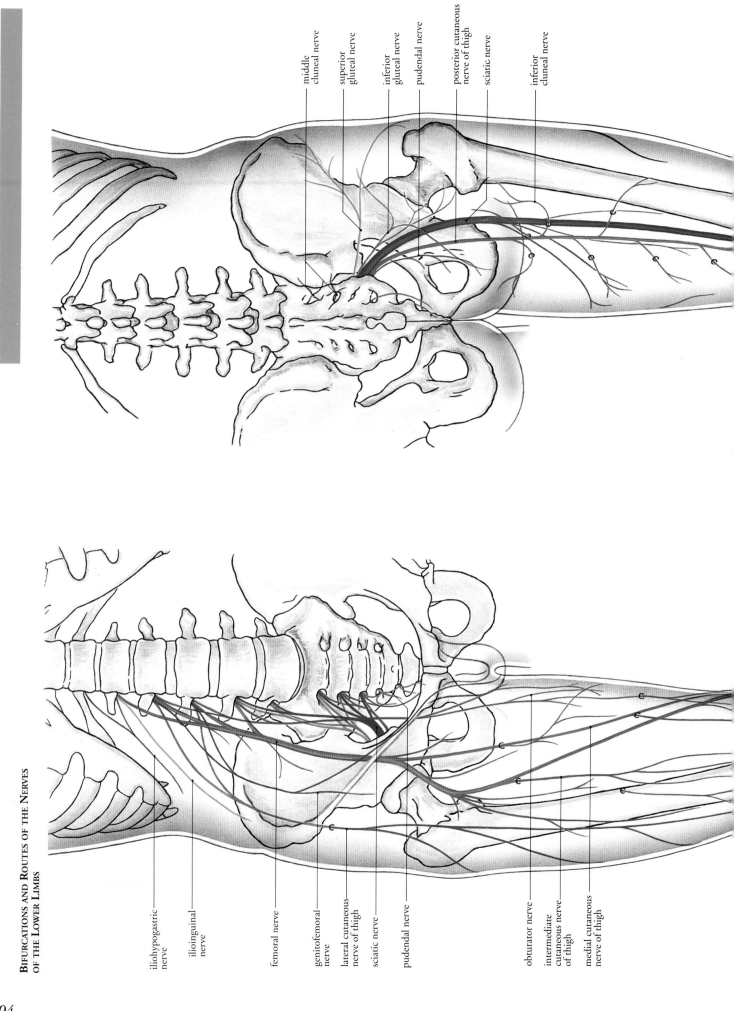

middle
cluneal nerve

superior
gluteal nerve

inferior
gluteal nerve

pudendal nerve

posterior cutaneous
nerve of thigh

sciatic nerve

inferior
cluneal nerve

BIFURCATIONS AND ROUTES OF THE NERVES
OF THE LOWER LIMBS

iliohypogastric
nerve

ilioinguinal
nerve

femoral nerve

genitofemoral
nerve

lateral cutaneous
nerve of thigh

sciatic nerve

pudendal nerve

obturator nerve

intermediate
cutaneous nerve
of thigh

medial cutaneous
nerve of thigh

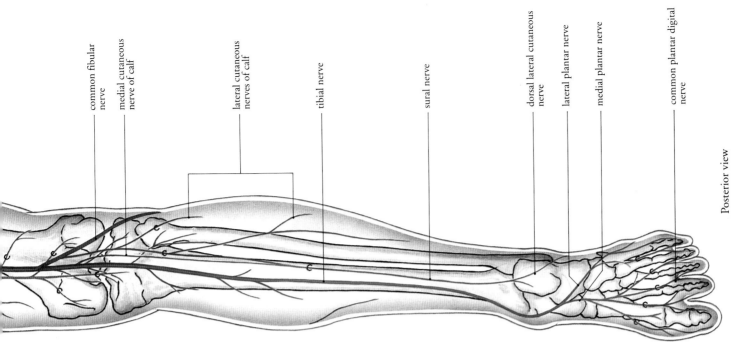

common fibular nerve

medial cutaneous nerve of calf

lateral cutaneous nerves of calf

tibial nerve

sural nerve

dorsal lateral cutaneous nerve

lateral plantar nerve

medial plantar nerve

common plantar digital nerve

Posterior view

Nerve Plexuses of the Lower Limbs. The nerves leading to the lower limbs extend from the lumbar nerve plexus and the sacral plexus. The nerves from the first through fourth lumbar vertebrae meet at the lumbar plexus. Branches extend into the muscles of the hips where they divide into the femoral, obturator, lateral femoral cutaneous, saphenous, genitofemoral, ilioinguinal, and iliohypogastric nerves. The sacral nerve plexus is the collection of the nerves of the fourth and fifth lumbar vertebrae and the sacral bone. Its branches include the sciatic, gluteal, and pudendal nerves. These nerves perform motor and sensory functions in the pelvic girdle and legs.

FEMORAL NERVE. The femoral nerve controls the pectineus sartorius, iliopsoas, and quadriceps muscles of the thigh. It branches into the anterior cutaneous nerve and the saphenous nerve. If the femoral nerve is paralyzed, the thigh cannot be extended or flexed, the upper body cannot be raised from a prone position, and it is not possible to climb stairs. Moreover, when standing or walking the knees can no longer maintain a fully extended position.

OBTURATOR NERVE. The obturator nerve controls the obturator muscle and the adductor muscles. If it is injured, the thighs cannot be closed and the injured leg cannot be crossed over the other leg.

SCIATIC NERVE. The sciatic nerve is the thickest nerve in the body. It divides at the distal end of the posterior thigh into the tibial and common fibular nerves. The sciatic nerve controls the flexor and adductor magnus muscles of the thigh and the flexors of the leg, foot, and toes. People with sciatic neuralgia feel sharp pain when extending the lower limb or when pressure is applied directly over the nerve.

COMMON FIBULAR NERVE. If the common fibular nerve is paralyzed, it results in dropping of the lateral edge and distal end of the foot.

Major Disorders: paralysis of the median nerve, paralysis of the ulnar nerve, paralysis of the radial nerve, paralysis of the brachial plexus, sciatic neuralgia, periodic paralysis, anterior tibial compartment syndrome.

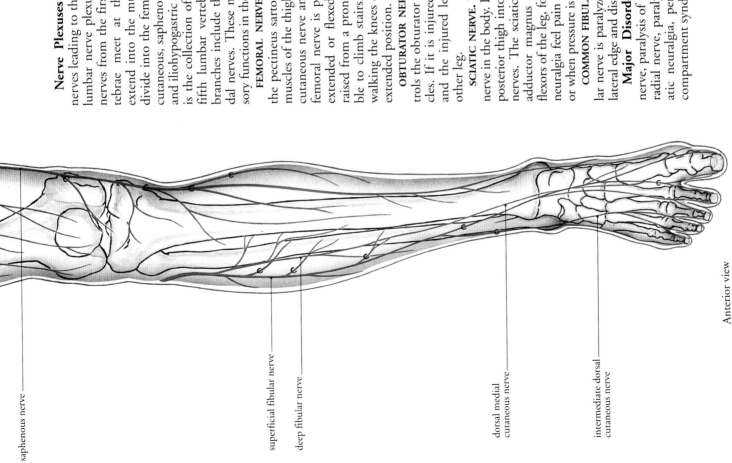

saphenous nerve

superficial fibular nerve

deep fibular nerve

dorsal medial cutaneous nerve

intermediate dorsal cutaneous nerve

Anterior view

5 The Human Body as a Whole

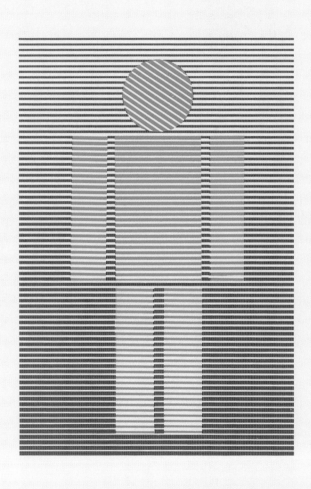

The Muscles

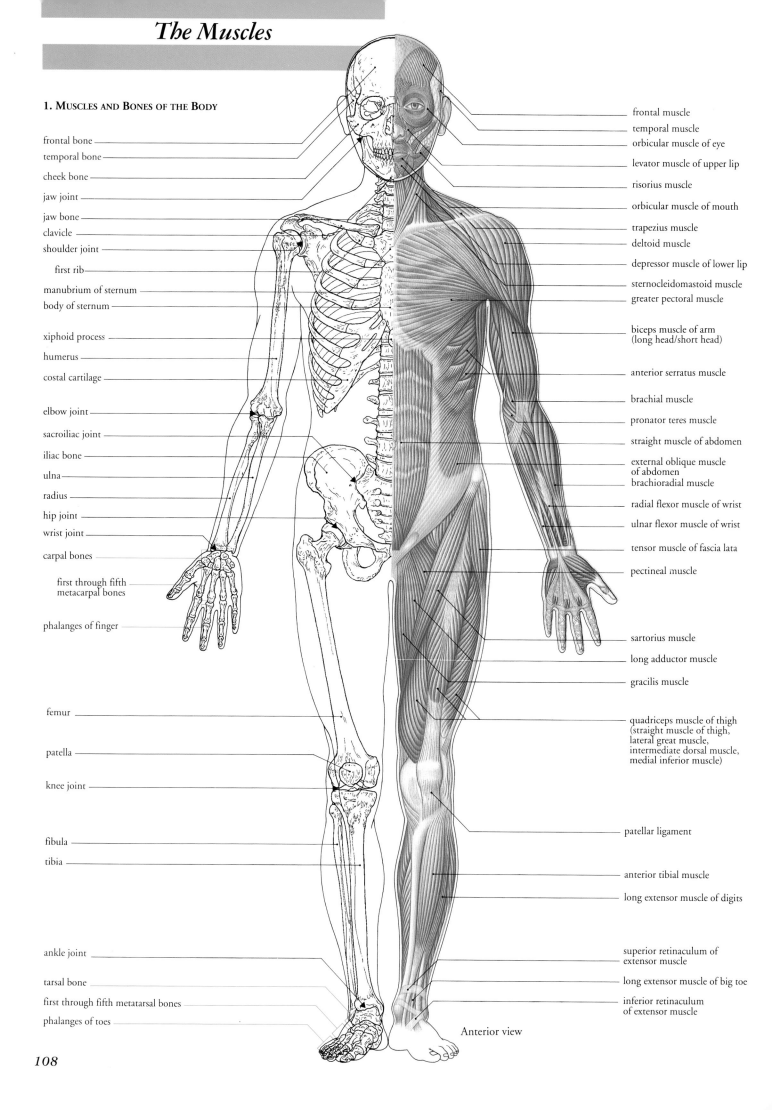

1. MUSCLES AND BONES OF THE BODY

frontal bone

temporal bone

cheek bone

jaw joint

jaw bone

clavicle

shoulder joint

first rib

manubrium of sternum

body of sternum

xiphoid process

humerus

costal cartilage

elbow joint

sacroiliac joint

iliac bone

ulna

radius

hip joint

wrist joint

carpal bones

first through fifth
metacarpal bones

phalanges of finger

femur

patella

knee joint

fibula

tibia

ankle joint

tarsal bone

first through fifth metatarsal bones

phalanges of toes

frontal muscle

temporal muscle

orbicular muscle of eye

levator muscle of upper lip

risorius muscle

orbicular muscle of mouth

trapezius muscle

deltoid muscle

depressor muscle of lower lip

sternocleidomastoid muscle

greater pectoral muscle

biceps muscle of arm
(long head/short head)

anterior serratus muscle

brachial muscle

pronator teres muscle

straight muscle of abdomen

external oblique muscle
of abdomen
brachioradial muscle

radial flexor muscle of wrist

ulnar flexor muscle of wrist

tensor muscle of fascia lata

pectineal muscle

sartorius muscle

long adductor muscle

gracilis muscle

quadriceps muscle of thigh
(straight muscle of thigh,
lateral great muscle,
intermediate dorsal muscle,
medial inferior muscle)

patellar ligament

anterior tibial muscle

long extensor muscle of digits

superior retinaculum of
extensor muscle

long extensor muscle of big toe

inferior retinaculum
of extensor muscle

Anterior view

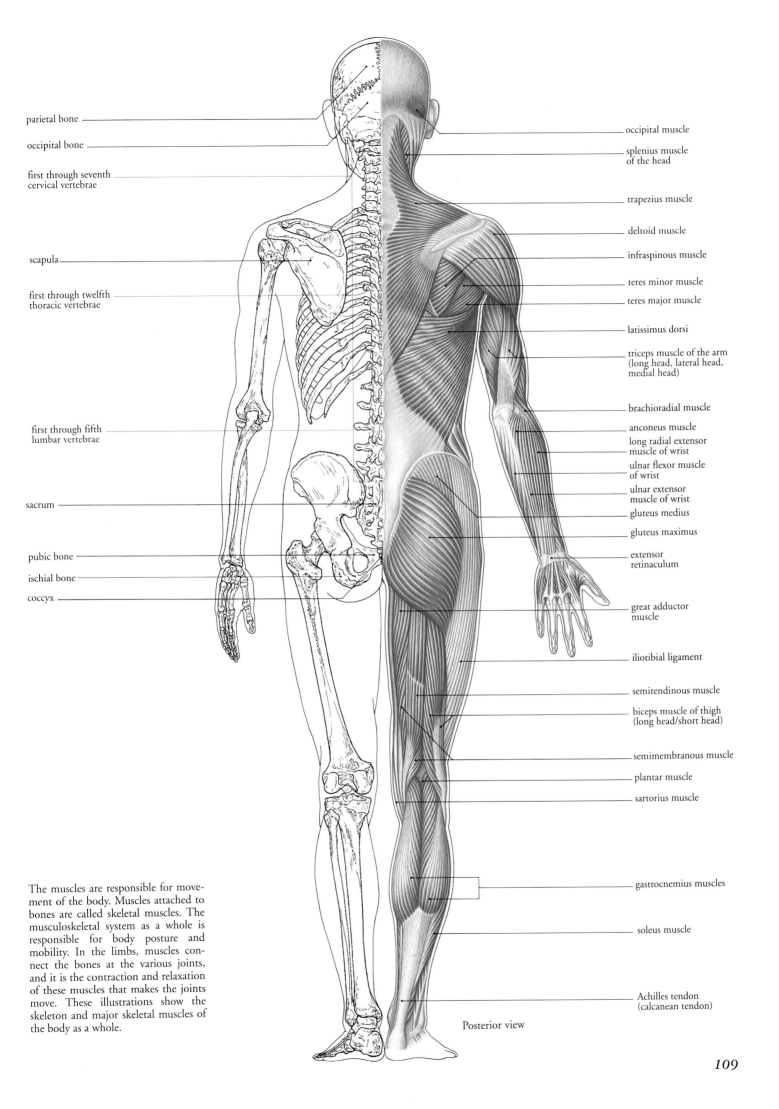

parietal bone

occipital bone

first through seventh
cervical vertebrae

scapula

first through twelfth
thoracic vertebrae

first through fifth
lumbar vertebrae

sacrum

pubic bone

ischial bone

coccyx

occipital muscle

splenius muscle
of the head

trapezius muscle

deltoid muscle

infraspinous muscle

teres minor muscle

teres major muscle

latissimus dorsi

triceps muscle of the arm
(long head, lateral head,
medial head)

brachioradial muscle

anconeus muscle

long radial extensor
muscle of wrist

ulnar flexor muscle
of wrist

ulnar extensor
muscle of wrist

gluteus medius

gluteus maximus

extensor
retinaculum

great adductor
muscle

iliotibial ligament

semitendinous muscle

biceps muscle of thigh
(long head/short head)

semimembranous muscle

plantar muscle

sartorius muscle

gastrocnemius muscles

soleus muscle

Achilles tendon
(calcanean tendon)

The muscles are responsible for movement of the body. Muscles attached to
bones are called skeletal muscles. The
musculoskeletal system as a whole is
responsible for body posture and
mobility. In the limbs, muscles connect the bones at the various joints,
and it is the contraction and relaxation
of these muscles that makes the joints
move. These illustrations show the
skeleton and major skeletal muscles of
the body as a whole.

Posterior view

109

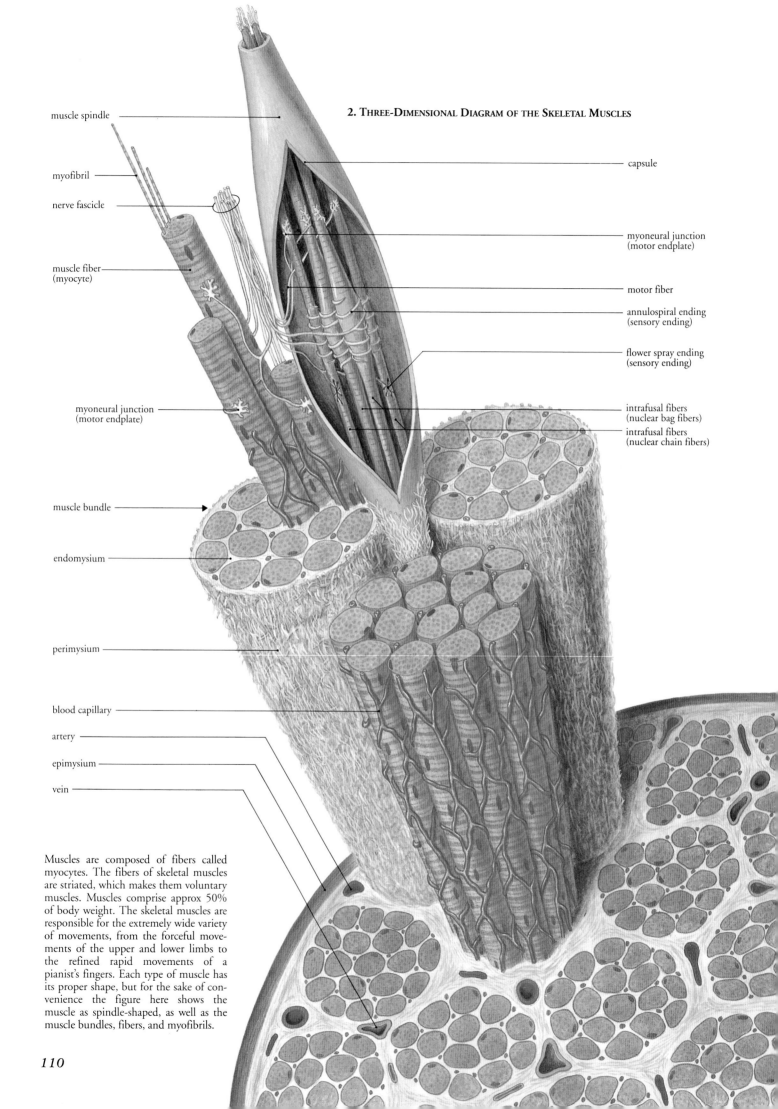

2. Three-Dimensional Diagram of the Skeletal Muscles

muscle spindle

myofibril

nerve fascicle

muscle fiber
(myocyte)

myoneural junction
(motor endplate)

muscle bundle

endomysium

perimysium

blood capillary

artery

epimysium

vein

capsule

myoneural junction
(motor endplate)

motor fiber

annulospiral ending
(sensory ending)

flower spray ending
(sensory ending)

intrafusal fibers
(nuclear bag fibers)

intrafusal fibers
(nuclear chain fibers)

Muscles are composed of fibers called myocytes. The fibers of skeletal muscles are striated, which makes them voluntary muscles. Muscles comprise approx 50% of body weight. The skeletal muscles are responsible for the extremely wide variety of movements, from the forceful movements of the upper and lower limbs to the refined rapid movements of a pianist's fingers. Each type of muscle has its proper shape, but for the sake of convenience the figure here shows the muscle as spindle-shaped, as well as the muscle bundles, fibers, and myofibrils.

3. STRUCTURE OF THE SMOOTH MUSCLES

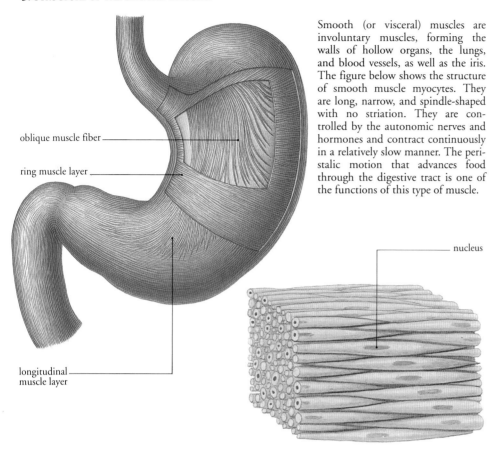

oblique muscle fiber

ring muscle layer

longitudinal muscle layer

nucleus

Smooth (or visceral) muscles are involuntary muscles, forming the walls of hollow organs, the lungs, and blood vessels, as well as the iris. The figure below shows the structure of smooth muscle myocytes. They are long, narrow, and spindle-shaped with no striation. They are controlled by the autonomic nerves and hormones and contract continuously in a relatively slow manner. The peristalic motion that advances food through the digestive tract is one of the functions of this type of muscle.

4. STRUCTURE OF THE CARDIAC MUSCLE

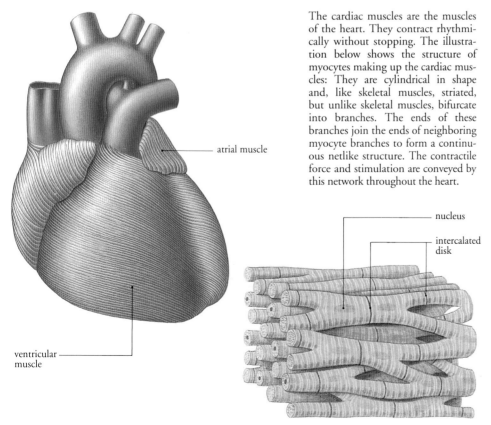

atrial muscle

ventricular muscle

nucleus

intercalated disk

The cardiac muscles are the muscles of the heart. They contract rhythmically without stopping. The illustration below shows the structure of myocytes making up the cardiac muscles: They are cylindrical in shape and, like skeletal muscles, striated, but unlike skeletal muscles, bifurcate into branches. The ends of these branches join the ends of neighboring myocyte branches to form a continuous netlike structure. The contractile force and stimulation are conveyed by this network throughout the heart.

Types of Muscles and Their Characteristics. The three types of muscles include striated, smooth, and cardiac muscles. Striated muscles (also called skeletal muscles) are attached to the skeleton and their functions include locomotion and movement, support, and the control of body openings. They can be contracted and relaxed at will, making them voluntary muscles. In contrast, the smooth muscles and cardiac muscles are involuntary muscles—cannot be moved at will. These muscles are controlled automatically by the autonomic nervous system.

For the most part, smooth muscles make up hollow organs, including the blood vessels, intestines, trachea, ureter, stomach, bladder, and the uterus. Compared with striated muscles, smooth muscles contract more slowly, tension does not increase with muscle expansion, and contraction is rhythmical. The cardiac muscles give shape to the heart and possess the features of both striated and smooth muscles.

Structure. STRIATED MUSCLES. Myocytes, the cells of muscle are long thin fibers. The nucleus is pushed toward the edge of the cell, and the sarcoplasm is made up mainly of myofibrils. Each muscle fiber is covered by a membrane called the endomysium. A collection of these fibers forms a muscle bundle (fasicle). The outside of each muscle bundle is covered by the perimysium, and a collection of these bundles is further covered by the epimysium and forms a muscle.

SMOOTH MUSCLES. Compared with striated muscles, smooth muscle fibers are smaller in diameter, shorter in length, and do not have striations.

CARDIAC MUSCLES. Cardiac muscle fibers are striated, but they are thinner and shorter than the fibers of skeletal muscles. Branches of cardiac muscle fibers join the branches of other cardiac muscle fibers so that they all respond as one when stimulated.

Function. A nerve impulse transmitted via motor nerve fibers reaches the junction of the nerve and muscle fibers (motor endplate or ganglionic terminal) and the striated muscle contracts. Fast-contracting muscles such as ocular muscles and the gastrocnemius muscles of the lower limbs have low levels of pigment (myoglobin) and are called "white muscles." These muscles contract rapidly but tire easily. Skeletal muscles rich in myoglobin are called "red muscles." These contract more slowly or continuously and tire less easily than do white muscles.

Major Disorders: muscular dystrophy, multiple myositis, myesthenia gravis, dermatomysitis, torticollis.

The Bones and Joints

1. Basic Structure of Bone

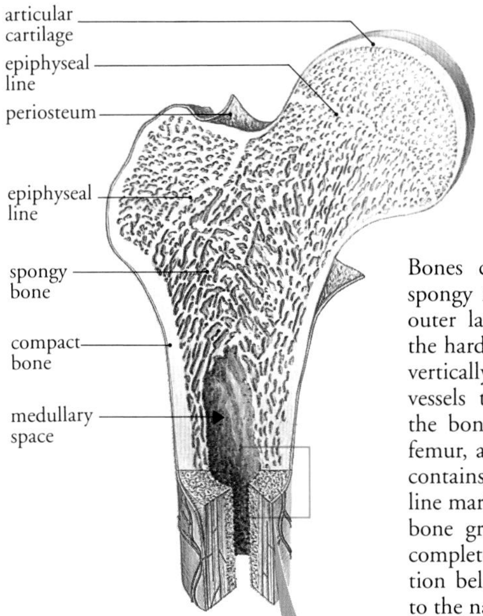

articular cartilage
epiphyseal line
periosteum
epiphyseal line
spongy bone
compact bone
medullary space

Bones consist of an inner layer of spongy matter, compact bone, and an outer layer called the periosteum. In the hard compact bone canals running vertically and horizontally house blood vessels that provide nourishment for the bone. In long bones such as the femur, a medullary canal in the center contains bone marrow. The epiphyseal line marks the cartilaginous layer where bone growth occurs. Once growth is complete this part ossifies. The illustration below shows bone as it is visible to the naked eye as well as the very fine structures as they may be viewed through a microscope.

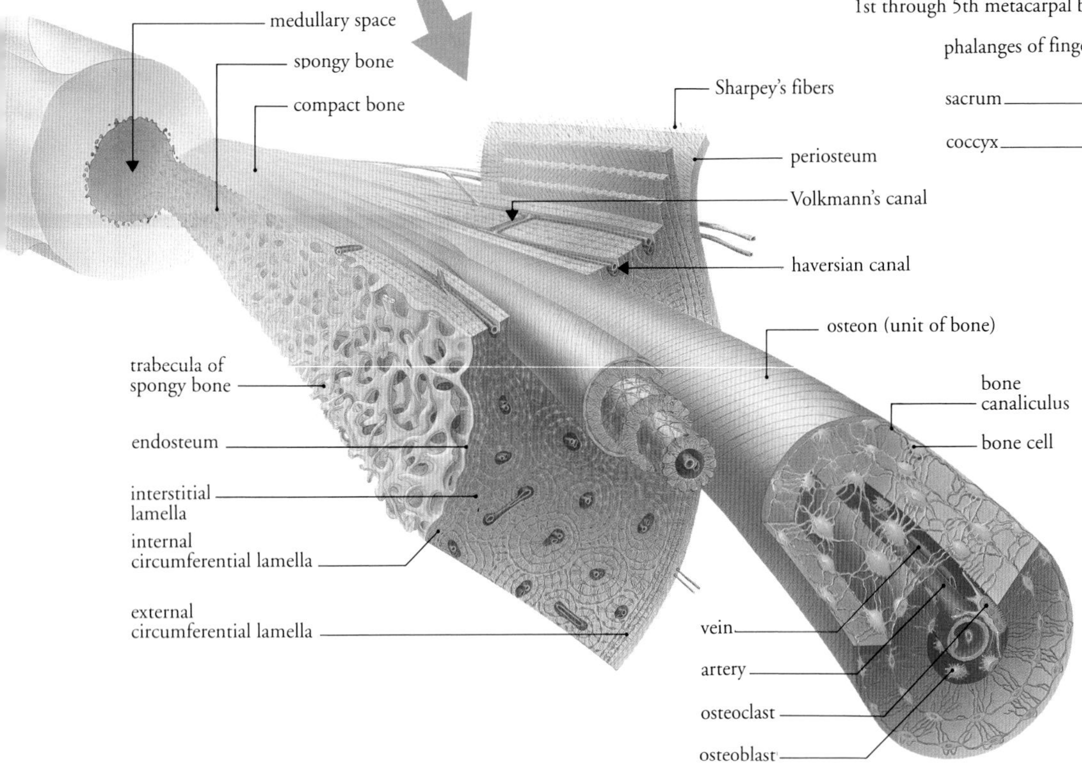

medullary space
spongy bone
compact bone

Sharpey's fibers
periosteum
Volkmann's canal
haversian canal
osteon (unit of bone)
bone canaliculus
bone cell

trabecula of spongy bone
endosteum
interstitial lamella
internal circumferential lamella
external circumferential lamella

vein
artery
osteoclast
osteoblast

2. Skeleton of the Body and Major Joints

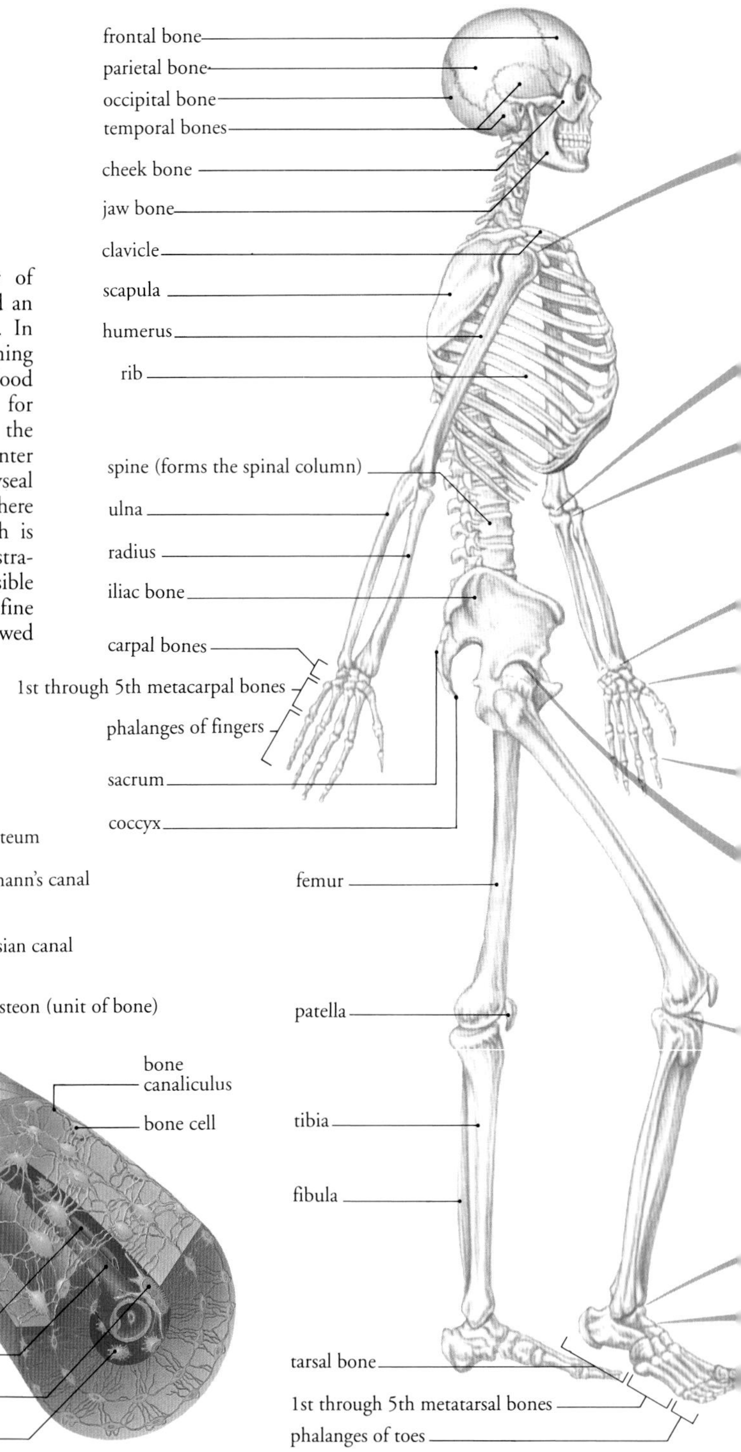

frontal bone
parietal bone
occipital bone
temporal bones
cheek bone
jaw bone
clavicle
scapula
humerus
rib
spine (forms the spinal column)
ulna
radius
iliac bone
carpal bones
1st through 5th metacarpal bones
phalanges of fingers
sacrum
coccyx
femur
patella
tibia
fibula
tarsal bone
1st through 5th metatarsal bones
phalanges of toes

BONE

Types. Bone is classified into five types by shape: long, short, flat, pneumatic, and mixed bone. The long bones are found in the limbs, and short bones are located in areas such as in the back of the hand (in the carpal region) and the foot (tarsal region). Flat bones are thin and flat, such as those that form the skull. Pneumatic bones have a hollow space, e.g., the maxilla (jaw). Mixed bones are flat bones that have a space within a thick section, e.g., the frontal bone of the skull.

Structure. BASIC STRUCTURE. The stem of tubular long bones and the outer part of short and flat bones are made of hard compact bone containing high levels of calcium phosphatase. The compact bone encloses the reticulated interior structure (spongy bone). The medullary canal is filled with marrow. Immediately after birth, the marrow produces red corpuscles (red marrow), but in the adult, the ability to produce red corpuscles diminishes and fatty material makes the marrow yellow in color.

FINE STRUCTURES. In the hard compact bone of long bones, structures that look like long green onions are bundled together vertically. Nerves and fine blood vessels pass through the center. Nourished by this rich flow of blood, bone destruction by osteo-

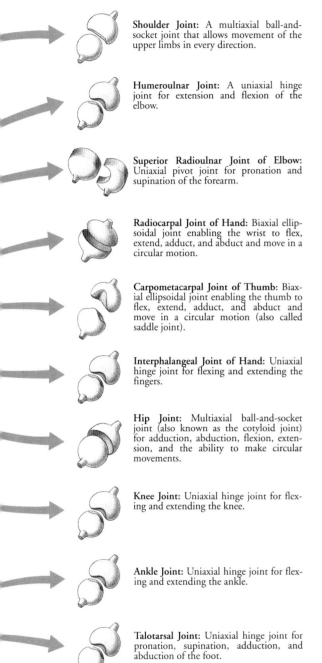

Shoulder Joint: A multiaxial ball-and-socket joint that allows movement of the upper limbs in every direction.

Humeroulnar Joint: A uniaxial hinge joint for extension and flexion of the elbow.

Superior Radioulnar Joint of Elbow: Uniaxial pivot joint for pronation and supination of the forearm.

Radiocarpal Joint of Hand: Biaxial ellipsoidal joint enabling the wrist to flex, extend, adduct, and abduct and move in a circular motion.

Carpometacarpal Joint of Thumb: Biaxial ellipsoidal joint enabling the thumb to flex, extend, adduct, and abduct and move in a circular motion (also called saddle joint).

Interphalangeal Joint of Hand: Uniaxial hinge joint for flexing and extending the fingers.

Hip Joint: Multiaxial ball-and-socket joint (also known as the cotyloid joint) for adduction, abduction, flexion, extension, and the ability to make circular movements.

Knee Joint: Uniaxial hinge joint for flexing and extending the knee.

Ankle Joint: Uniaxial hinge joint for flexing and extending the ankle.

Talotarsal Joint: Uniaxial hinge joint for pronation, supination, adduction, and abduction of the foot.

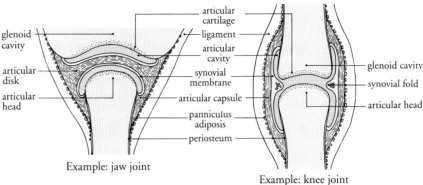

Example: jaw joint

Example: knee joint

The basic structure of a joint includes an articular head that fits in a cavity, which is covered by tissue called the articular capsule. The surfaces facing each other are wrapped by smooth articular cartilage and the inside of the articular capsule is covered by a synovial membrane, which excretes a lubricating mucus (synovial fluid) that enables the joint to move smoothly. In the articular cavity, synovial folds (the knee) or an articular disk (the mandibular joint) function to facilitate smooth movement.

Joints

Types. Joints are divided into three types, uniaxial, biaxial, and multiaxial, based on the number of axes present.

A uniaxial joint has only one axis and is able to flex and extend. A biaxial joint, such as the wrist joint, has axes going in two directions that intersect at right angles. The wrist joint allows the hand to move in a circle. However, the wrist cannot rotate around the axis, i.e., it cannot abduct and adduct in a twisting motion if the wrist is in a fixed position. A multiaxial joint like the shoulder has numerous axes, making movement possible in every direction.

Types by Shape of Articular Surface. Joints can be divided into four types based on the shape of the articular surface.

A ball-and-socket joint has a round head that fits in the round hollow of a cavity, enabling movement in every direction. It is a multiaxial joint.

The radiocarpal joint of the hand is an ellipsoidal joint. The articular surface is oval in shape, permitting biaxial movement along the long and short axes.

A hinge joint is a uniaxial joint exemplified by the elbow and knee, which can flex or extend only on one plane, like the hinge of a door.

A pivot joint is also uniaxial, but because the articular surfaces resemble the relationship between the wheel and axle of a car, it is able to rotate like a wheel about the central axis. The radioulnar joint of the forearm is a pivot joint that enables the palm of the hand to be turned forward (supination) and backward (pronation).

One type of ellipsoidal joint is a saddle joint, which moves the thumb. Besides flexion and extension along two axes this joint allows the thumb to come in contact with the other fingers of the hand. It also permits the tip of the thumb to be raised when the palm is facing upward.

clasts and bone production by osteoblasts takes place continuously. This constant replenishment ensures that the structure is well suited mechanically to meet the demands made by the pressure applied to bone.

Function. The bones are the framework that supports the body's structure and they protect the brain and other organs from trauma. Bone marrow produces corpuscles (red corpuscles and white corpuscles such as granulocytes and monocytes) and acts as the storehouse for calcium, which plays an important role in the functioning of the body.

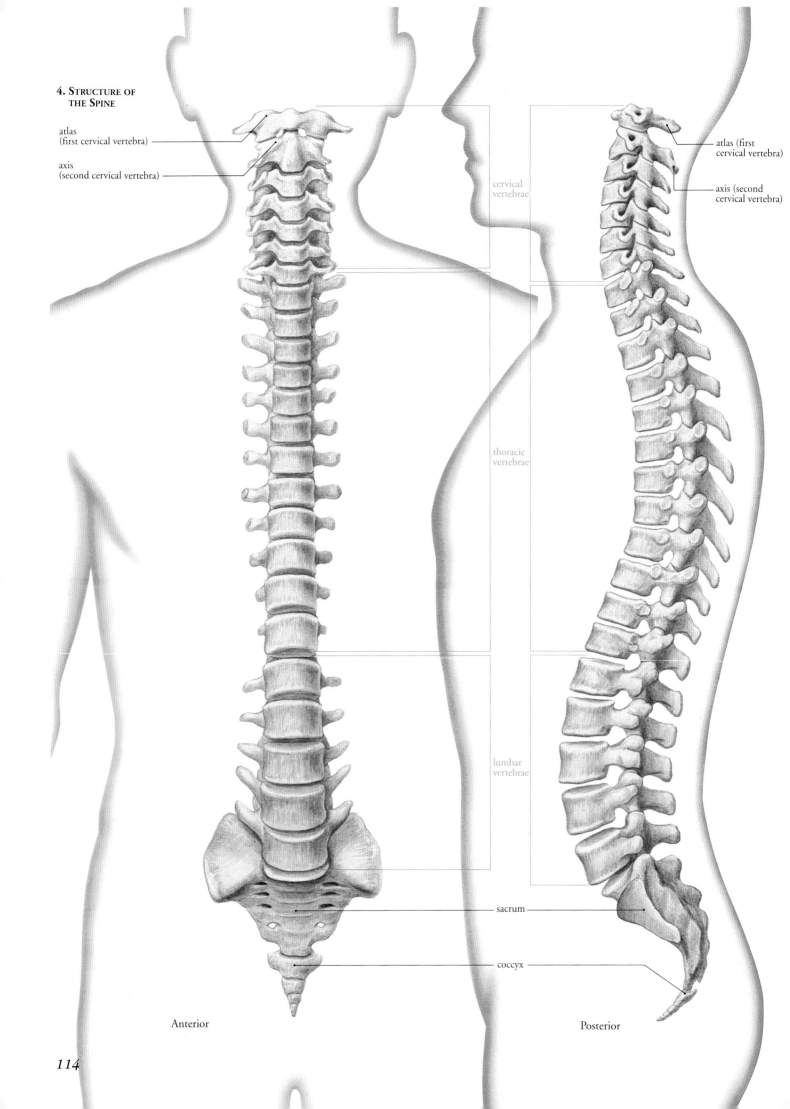

4. STRUCTURE OF THE SPINE

atlas
(first cervical vertebra)

axis
(second cervical vertebra)

cervical
vertebrae

atlas (first
cervical vertebra)

axis (second
cervical vertebra)

thoracic
vertebrae

lumbar
vertebrae

sacrum

coccyx

Anterior

Posterior

5. STRUCTURE OF THE LUMBAR VERTEBRAE

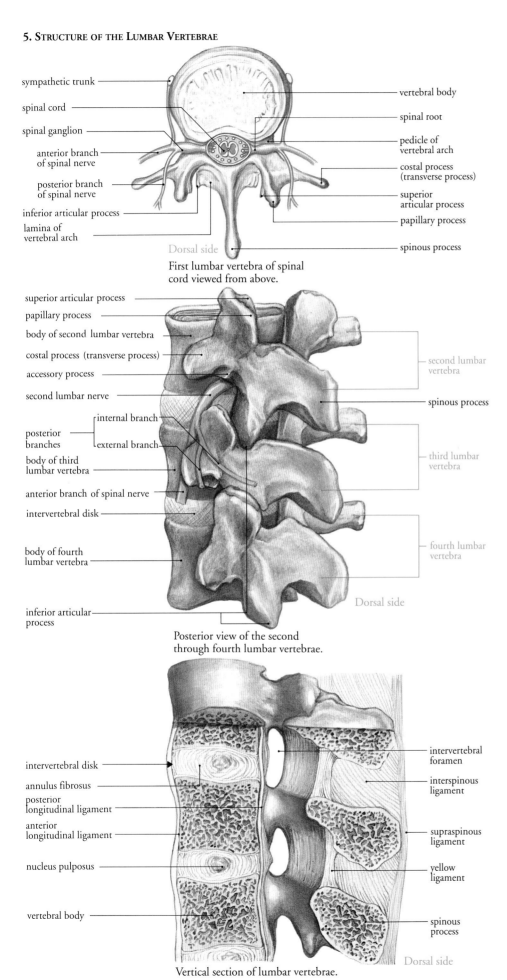

sympathetic trunk

spinal cord

spinal ganglion

anterior branch
of spinal nerve

posterior branch
of spinal nerve

inferior articular process

lamina of
vertebral arch

vertebral body

spinal root

pedicle of
vertebral arch

costal process
(transverse process)

superior
articular process

papillary process

spinous process

Dorsal side

First lumbar vertebra of spinal
cord viewed from above.

superior articular process

papillary process

body of second lumbar vertebra

costal process (transverse process)

accessory process

second lumbar nerve

posterior
branches
  internal branch
  external branch

body of third
lumbar vertebra

anterior branch of spinal nerve

intervertebral disk

body of fourth
lumbar vertebra

inferior articular
process

second lumbar
vertebra

spinous process

third lumbar
vertebra

fourth lumbar
vertebra

Dorsal side

Posterior view of the second
through fourth lumbar vertebrae.

intervertebral disk

annulus fibrosus

posterior
longitudinal ligament

anterior
longitudinal ligament

nucleus pulposus

vertebral body

intervertebral
foramen

interspinous
ligament

supraspinous
ligament

yellow
ligament

spinous
process

Dorsal side

Vertical section of lumbar vertebrae.

6. CONDITION OF HERNIATED DISK

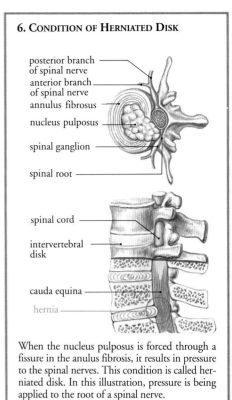

posterior branch
of spinal nerve

anterior branch
of spinal nerve

annulus fibrosus

nucleus pulposus

spinal ganglion

spinal root

spinal cord

intervertebral
disk

cauda equina

hernia

When the nucleus pulposus is forced through a fissure in the anulus fibrosis, it results in pressure to the spinal nerves. This condition is called herniated disk. In this illustration, pressure is being applied to the root of a spinal nerve.

SPINAL COLUMN

Structure. The spinal column is made up of 26 bones: 24 uniquely shaped vertebrae plus the sacrum and the tail bone (coccyx), which are located at the end of the backbone. Between each vertebra is a "cushion" called an intervertebral disk. On the anterior side of each vertebra is the vertebral body, which is in the shape of an oval disk. On the posterior side of each vertebra is an opening (vertebral foramen) through which the spinal cord passes. Surrounding this opening is the vertebral arch; on the posterior side of the vertebral arch are the spinous process, and the left and right transverse processes. Each transverse process has an articular process above and below.

The 24 vertebrae include 7 cervical vertebrae, 12 thoracic vertebrae, and 5 lumbar vertebrae.

Function and Characteristics. When the spinal column is viewed from the back it appears to be straight, but from the side it can be seen that it is curved in the shape of the letter "S." This curve functions to support the head, which is heavy. The vertebral foramen within the vertebral arch form a vertical passage to hold the spinal cord. The number of vertebrae that make up the spinal column depends on the species of animal. In four-footed animals, the size of the vertebral bodies does not vary much, and the curve of the spine is simpler.

Major Disorders: osteoporosis, osteomalacia, arthritis, herniated disk, osteoarthritis, spondylolysis, spondylolisthesis.

The Skin and Hair

1. Structure of the Skin

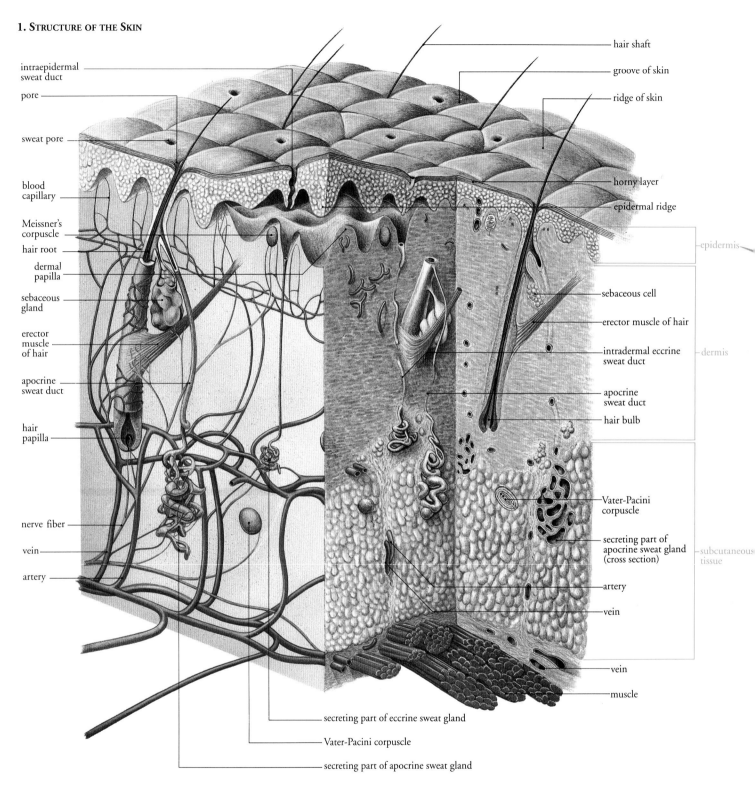

intraepidermal sweat duct

pore

sweat pore

blood capillary

Meissner's corpuscle

hair root

dermal papilla

sebaceous gland

erector muscle of hair

apocrine sweat duct

hair papilla

nerve fiber

vein

artery

hair shaft

groove of skin

ridge of skin

horny layer

epidermal ridge

epidermis

sebaceous cell

erector muscle of hair

intradermal eccrine sweat duct

apocrine sweat duct

hair bulb

dermis

Vater-Pacini corpuscle

secreting part of apocrine sweat gland (cross section)

artery

vein

vein

muscle

subcutaneous tissue

secreting part of eccrine sweat gland

Vater-Pacini corpuscle

secreting part of apocrine sweat gland

SKIN

Skin covers all body surfaces. In an adult male it is approx 1.8 sq m and weighs approx 4.8 kg, or approx 8.8% of total body weight.

Structure. Skin is composed of an outer layer called the epidermis and an inner layer called the dermis. The term "skin" often includes the structures found in the subcutaneous tissue, such as the sweat glands, sebaceous glands, hair roots and follicles, blood vessels, lymphatic vessels, and peripheral nerves.

EPIDERMIS. The palms of the hands and the soles of the feet (including the toes and fingers) include a horny layer of skin that is over 1 mm thick. Elsewhere, however, the skin is only approx 0.1–0.2 mm thick. Under the horny layer are the granular layer, spiny layer, and basal layer. The columnar cells of the basal layer divide continuously to form new cells, which push their way to the surface. It takes 2 wk for these cells to reach the granular layer and an additional 2 wk to reach the horny layer. After 4 wk they flake and peel off.

DERMIS. The dermis is divided into a papillary layer, subpapillary layer, and reticular layer. The most numerous fibers in the dermis are collagen fibers; these are covered by elastic and reticular fibers.

2. KERATINIZATION OF THE SKIN

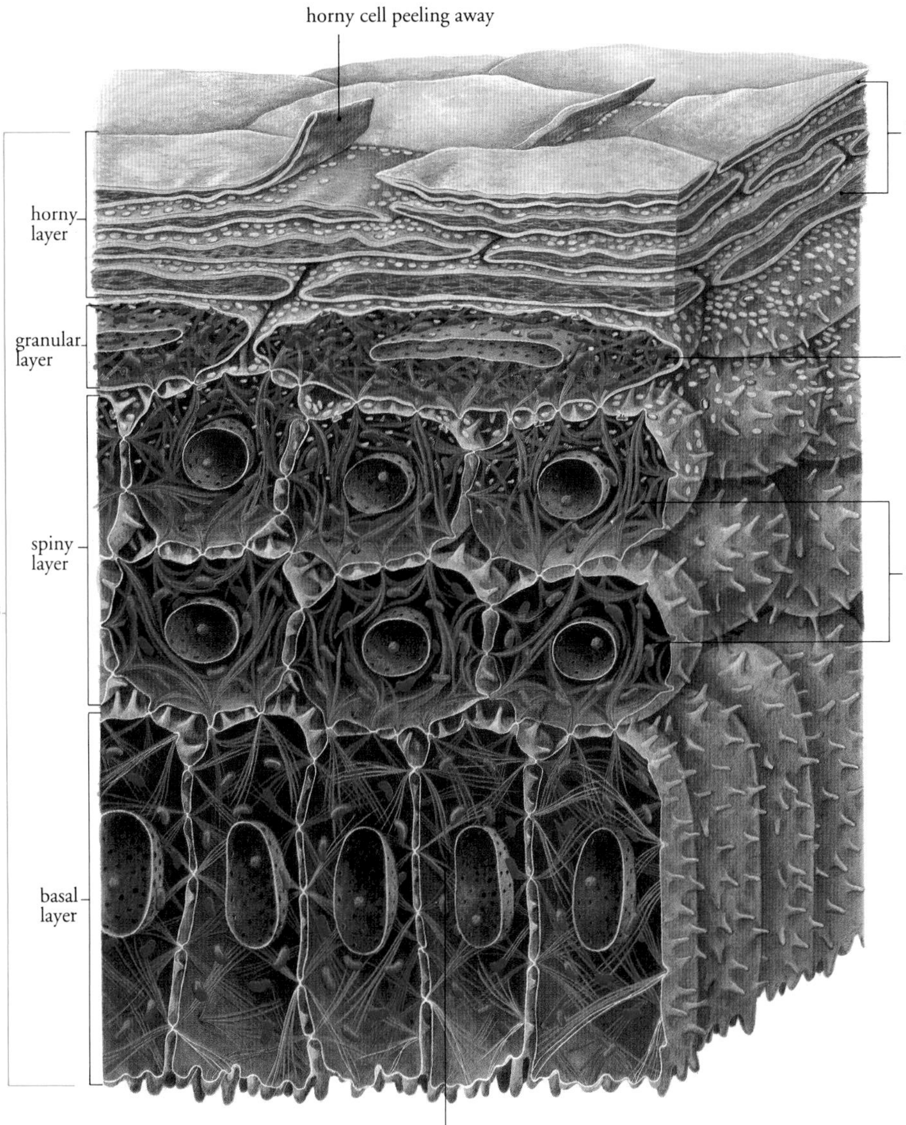

horny cell peeling away

horny cells

horny layer

granular layer

spiny layer

basal layer

ermis

granular cell

prickle cells

basal cell (columnar cell)

As a result of division of the columnar cells of the basal layer of the epidermis, young cells proliferate and push their way toward the surface, forming the spiny and granular layers. At the surface, they lose their nuclei and form the horny layer. After a time the horny layer flakes and peels away.

3. SURFACE OF SKIN VIEWED BY A SCANNING ELECTRON MICROSCOPE

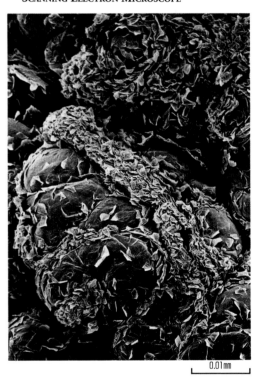

0.01 mm

What look like dry leaves are horny cells that have keratinized and are peeling off.

ACCESSORY ORGANS OF THE SKIN. Sebaceous glands secrete sebum at the hair roots to cover the surface of hair and epidermis with an oily film. Apocrine sweat glands produce a complex secretion with a strong odor and are numerous in certain areas of the body, such as under the arms and in the genital region. Eccrine sweat glands are distributed throughout the entire epidermis but are particularly numerous in the palms of the hands and soles of the feet.

Skin Color. Approximately 5–10% of the cells of the basal layer produce the pigment melanin, which is incorporated in the epithelial cells. The color of the skin differs depending on the amount of melanin in the cells.

Function. The skin provides powerful protection, guarding the body against physical forces such as heat, cold, sunrays, friction, pressure, and various chemicals. It is also a sensory receptor that senses pain, touch, and temperature. The sweat glands produce perspiration in response to emotional stimulation and to adjust body temperature.

Major Disorders: atopic dermatitis, scabies, dyshidrosis, athlete's foot, acne vulgaris, chilblain.

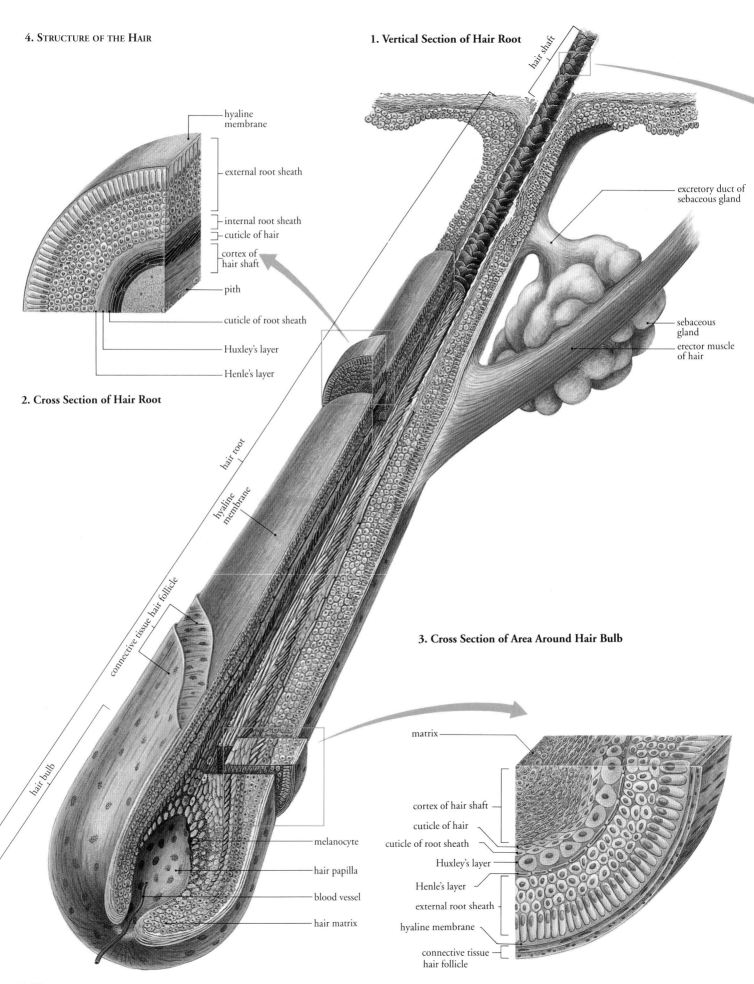

4. STRUCTURE OF THE HAIR

1. Vertical Section of Hair Root

hair shaft

hyaline membrane

external root sheath

internal root sheath

cuticle of hair

cortex of hair shaft

pith

cuticle of root sheath

Huxley's layer

Henle's layer

2. Cross Section of Hair Root

excretory duct of sebaceous gland

sebaceous gland

erector muscle of hair

hair root

hyaline membrane

connective tissue hair follicle

hair bulb

3. Cross Section of Area Around Hair Bulb

matrix

cortex of hair shaft

cuticle of hair

cuticle of root sheath

Huxley's layer

Henle's layer

external root sheath

hyaline membrane

connective tissue hair follicle

melanocyte

hair papilla

blood vessel

hair matrix

4. Section of Hair Shaft

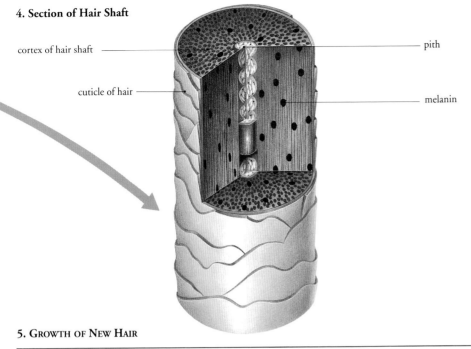

cortex of hair shaft — — pith

cuticle of hair — — melanin

5. Growth of New Hair

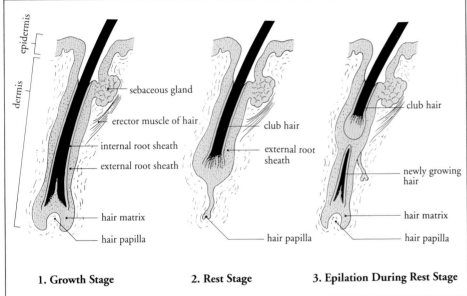

epidermis

dermis

sebaceous gland

erector muscle of hair

internal root sheath

external root sheath

club hair

external root sheath

club hair

newly growing hair

hair matrix

hair matrix

hair matrix

hair papilla

hair papilla

hair papilla

1. Growth Stage — **2. Rest Stage** — **3. Epilation During Rest Stage**

6. Scalp and Head Hair Viewed by Scanning Electron Microscope

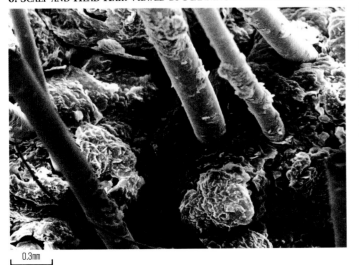

0.3mm

The bulb of the hair swells during the growth stage. The cells of the hair matrix located in the bulb actively divide to make hair grow. At the end of a hair root in the rest stage is a keratinous process that grows between the cells of the hair follicle. The length of the hair root in the rest stage is one-half to two-thirds that in the growth stage. Hair in the rest stage will eventually fall out.

Hair growing from the scalp. Dandruff accumulates at the root.

Hair

Hair is derived from the keratin of skin. Although the physiologic functions of hair include acting as a sensory agent, protecting the scalp, and retaining heat, it also has strong aesthetic significance among humans.

Structure. The part of the hair protruding from the surface of the skin is the hair shaft. The root lies buried approx 4–5 mm in the skin, and the base of the root is covered by the follicle. During the growth stage the root end of the hair is swollen and round, resembling a flask in shape; in the rest stage, the swelling disappears, and the root looks like a stick. Matrix is found in the center of a hair and is covered by the cortex and cuticle. A cross section of the straight hair of Asians is circular in shape, whereas that of the wavy hair of Caucasians is oval, and that of the tight curls of Blacks is shaped like a kidney bean. Located near the hair roots, erector muscles make hair stand up. Nearby, sebaceous glands secrete an oily substance that covers the hair.

Growth Stage and Rest Stage. Hair follicles undergo alternating periods of a growth (lasting from 2–5 yr) and a rest (lasting 3–4 mo). During the active stage hair grows at a rate of about 0.3–0.5 mm per d, and in the rest stage it falls out. The reason humans have long hair is not because it grows fast but because the active stage is long and the rest stage is short.

Hair Color. Hair color is determined by the type of melanin pigment in the cortex and by the amount of air taken in by the hair. If a lot of black melanin is present, then the hair is black. An abundance of air in the hairs result in white hair.

Type. The hair that grows on the head—long hair—grows naturally to a length of 10 mm or more. The hair that does not grow to that length is called short hair. Short hair is classified into asexual hair, which does not change after puberty, sexual hair common to both sexes (underarm hair, lower half of pubic hair), and male hair (chest hair, upper half of pubic hair).

Thickness. In humans the only skin without hair is found on the palms of the hands, the soles of the feet, the backs of the tips of the fingers, the red part of the lips, and the glans, foreskin, and clitoris. Individual thickness varies significantly, but scalp hair is usually thickest, with about 100,000 in the adult.

Major Disorders: alopecia areata, alopecia prematura.

The Blood and Lymph

Blood nourishes the cells that make up the body, whereas lymph serves to prevent infection by pathogens.

Size of the Circulatory System. The blood vessels in the adult human take up approx 3% of the total body weight; they are approx 90,000 km long, and the surface area within the vessels is as high as 6300 sq m. The amount of blood in the normal adult is equivalent to approx 1/13 total body weight.

Pulmonary and Systemic Circulations of Blood. Blood is moved by the contractions of the heart through the arteries, circulating from the lungs all the way to the capillaries, where gas exchange and metabolism occur. After this has been accomplished, the blood collects in the veins and returns to the heart.

Pulmonary Circulation. Venous blood exits by the right ventricle of the heart, passes through the pulmonary artery, and enters the lungs, where gas exchange replenishes oxygen and the blood becomes arterial blood. This blood then returns to the heart through the two left pulmonary veins and two right pulmonary veins. This means that venous blood flows through the arteries and arterial blood flows through the veins in pulmonary circulation.

Systemic Circulation. Arterial blood that has returned from the lungs to the left atrium of the heart exits from the left ventricle through the aorta to the body. Right outside the heart (at the aortic arch) three arteries branch off toward the upper part of the body. These branches reach to every corner of the upper body, including the head and arms. The artery leading toward the lower half of the body becomes the descending aorta (thoracic aorta, abdominal aorta) before branching off toward various organs and the lower limbs. Each artery branches out into very fine arterioles and capillaries. The venous blood then collects in veins that become larger and larger, forming the superior and inferior vena cava and coronary sinus (the opening through which blood that has nourished the cardiac muscles returns). The blood then returns to the right atrium of the heart.

Flow of Lymph. Lymph flows out from capillaries and collects in the lymphatic vessels. Lymphatic vessels are distributed throughout the entire body in close concert with the veins. Lymphatic vessels begin as small capillaries and become major passages such as the thoracic duct. These vessels empty into the vein at the base of the neck. The lymphatic fluid inside is transported by body action such as muscle contraction. Lymph nodes, which act as filters for lymph, are located throughout the body.

1. DISTRIBUTION OF ARTERIES THROUGHOUT THE BODY

1. Arterial Routes

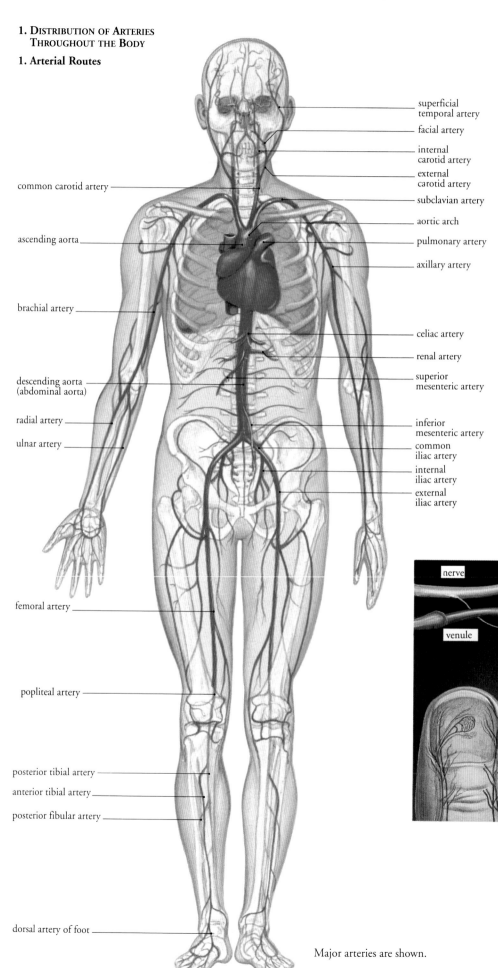

common carotid artery

ascending aorta

brachial artery

descending aorta (abdominal aorta)

radial artery

ulnar artery

femoral artery

popliteal artery

posterior tibial artery

anterior tibial artery

posterior fibular artery

dorsal artery of foot

superficial temporal artery

facial artery

internal carotid artery

external carotid artery

subclavian artery

aortic arch

pulmonary artery

axillary artery

celiac artery

renal artery

superior mesenteric artery

inferior mesenteric artery

common iliac artery

internal iliac artery

external iliac artery

nerve

venule

Major arteries are shown.

2. Places Where Blood Pulse Can Be Felt from Outside the Body

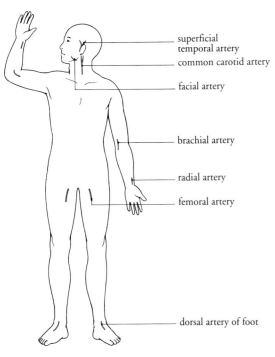

superficial temporal artery

common carotid artery

facial artery

brachial artery

radial artery

femoral artery

dorsal artery of foot

These arteries are located just beneath the skin, so a pulse can be felt at these places. Moreover, the arteries here are situated over hard tissue such as bone, so if bleeding occurs below the pulse point, it can be stopped by pressing on the artery above the injury.

3. How the Arteries and Veins Connect

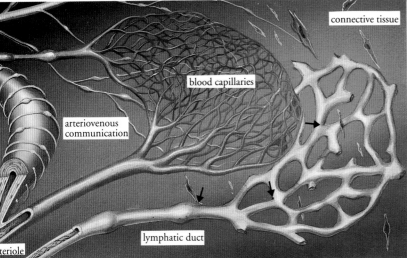

connective tissue

blood capillaries

arteriovenous communication

lymphatic duct

arteriole

This illustration shows arteriovenous communication and capillaries. In general, arteries gradually become thinner, forming arterioles and then capillaries; the capillaries then turn into venules. In some places, however (e.g., the mucous membrane lining the esophagus, the skin, and the tips of the fingers), arterioles and venules connect directly with each other. This is known as arteriovenous communication.

Capillaries are passages formed by a certain type of cell (endothelial), and a plasmalike fluid (indicated by arrows) seeps out from the joints. This substance flows between the cells and becomes (liquid) lymph. Lymph collects in lymphatic vessels, which gradually flow into larger and larger vessels until finally most lymph enters the veins.

2. Distribution of Veins and Lymphatic Vessels Throughout the Body

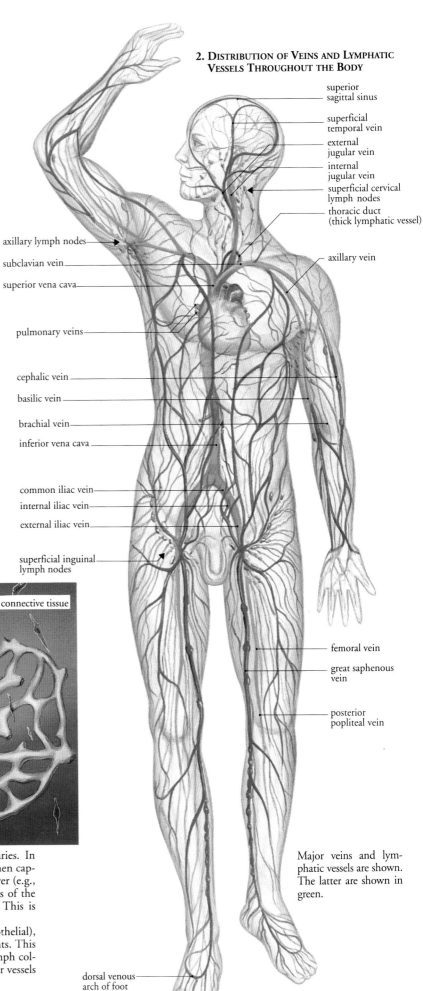

superior sagittal sinus

superficial temporal vein

external jugular vein

internal jugular vein

superficial cervical lymph nodes

thoracic duct (thick lymphatic vessel)

axillary vein

axillary lymph nodes

subclavian vein

superior vena cava

pulmonary veins

cephalic vein

basilic vein

brachial vein

inferior vena cava

common iliac vein

internal iliac vein

external iliac vein

superficial inguinal lymph nodes

femoral vein

great saphenous vein

posterior popliteal vein

dorsal venous arch of foot

Major veins and lymphatic vessels are shown. The latter are shown in green.

121

Duality of Circulation. Duality of circulation is observed in the liver, lung, and kidney. In the liver, the hepatic artery supplies oxygen and the portal vein delivers nutrients from the digestive tract to the liver. In the lung, the pulmonary arteries transport venous blood to the alveoli for gas exchange and the tracheal arteries supply nourishment to the lung itself. In the kidney, the renal arteries become capillaries in both the glomeruli and convoluted tubules, where crude urine is filtered and oxygen and nutrients are supplied to the kidney.

Structure of Blood Vessels. ARTERIES. The wall of an artery is made up of three layers: the tunica externa, tunica media, and tunica interna. Depending on the structure of the wall, arteries are divided into three types: elastic arteries, which have numerous elastic fibers in the tunica media, muscular arteries, which have few elastic fibers but many muscle fibers, and a third type that is a combination of the two. The inner side of the tunica interna is lined with a layer of endothelial cells, which have a smooth surface. The tunica media is a layer of smooth muscles arranged in rings; these muscles are a combination of elastic fibers and muscle fibers. In the muscular type of artery, instead of an internal elastic membrane (internal elastic lamina), numerous layers of elastic lamina overlap on the inner side of the tunica media. The Tunica externa is made of durable connective tissue. Blood vessels supplying nutrients are found on the outer side of the tunica externa and tunica media.

VEINS. Like arteries, veins have three layers: the tunica interna, tunica media, and tunica externa. The two types of veins include subfascial veins (which have a thin wall and little elasticity), and epifascial veins (which have many elastic fibers in the tunica media and tunica externa). Pairs of semicircular valves within the vessels prevent backflow of blood to the extremities. Venous valves are found in the arms and legs but not in the veins of the head, neck, or torso.

Circulation in the Fetus. Circulation in a fetus differs from circulation in a neonate. The characteristic feature of fetal circulation is the absence of a pulmonary circulation, so gas exchange as well as nutrition and waste removal occur in the placenta (see page 85, Figure 5). Two umbilical arteries transport the venous blood from the fetus to the placenta, whereas umbilical veins deliver arterial blood from the placenta to the fetus. Pulmonary circulation begins with the newborn's first cries after delivery.

Major Disorders: arteriosclerosis, phlebeurysm, hypertension, leukemia.

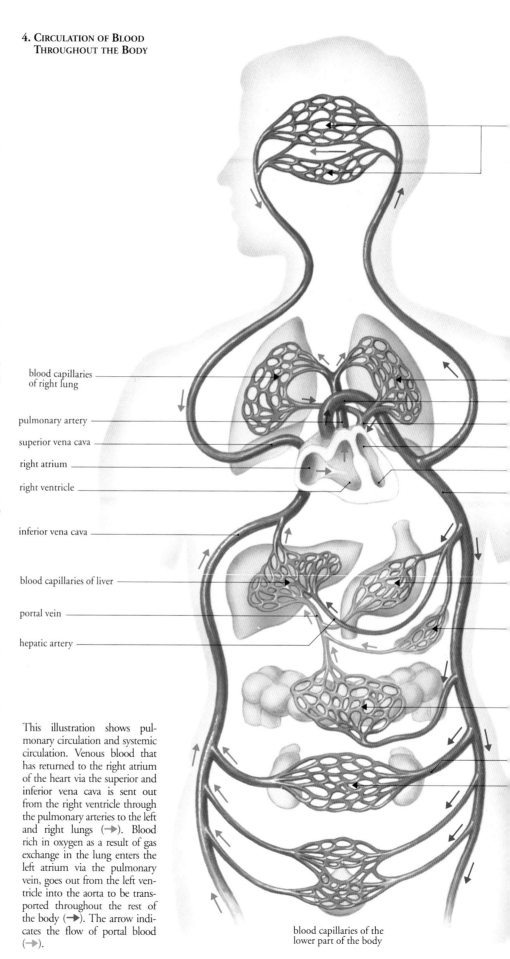

4. CIRCULATION OF BLOOD THROUGHOUT THE BODY

blood capillaries of right lung

pulmonary artery

superior vena cava

right atrium

right ventricle

inferior vena cava

blood capillaries of liver

portal vein

hepatic artery

This illustration shows pulmonary circulation and systemic circulation. Venous blood that has returned to the right atrium of the heart via the superior and inferior vena cava is sent out from the right ventricle through the pulmonary arteries to the left and right lungs (→). Blood rich in oxygen as a result of gas exchange in the lung enters the left atrium via the pulmonary vein, goes out from the left ventricle into the aorta to be transported throughout the rest of the body (→). The arrow indicates the flow of portal blood (→).

blood capillaries of the lower part of the body

5. STRUCTURE OF THE BLOOD VESSEL

1. Structure of the Arterial Wall

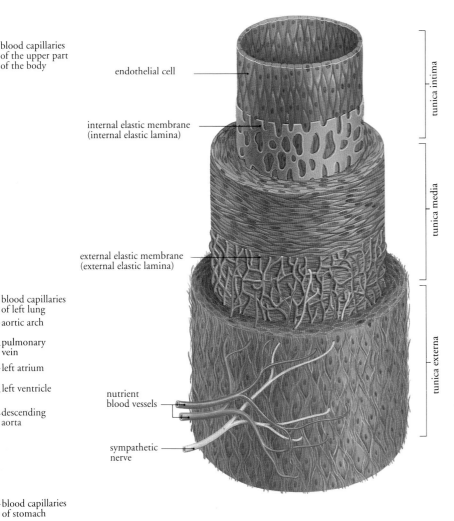

blood capillaries of the upper part of the body

endothelial cell

internal elastic membrane (internal elastic lamina)

tunica intima

external elastic membrane (external elastic lamina)

tunica media

blood capillaries of left lung

aortic arch

pulmonary vein

left atrium

left ventricle

descending aorta

nutrient blood vessels

tunica externa

sympathetic nerve

blood capillaries of stomach

blood capillaries of spleen

blood capillaries of intestine

renal artery

blood capillaries of kidneys

2. Difference Between the Wall of Artery and the Wall of Vein

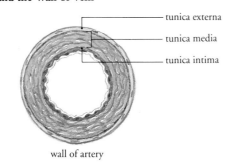

tunica externa

tunica media

tunica intima

wall of artery

tunica externa

tunica media

tunica intima

wall of vein

Because the arteries must take in blood sent out by strong pressure from the heart they have thicker walls than veins. The arterial walls are also flexible and have good elasticity.

3. Circulation of Blood in Veins and Operation of the Valves

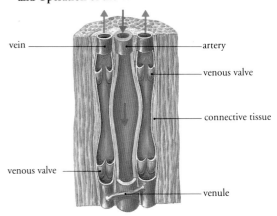

vein

artery

venous valve

connective tissue

venous valve

venule

This illustration shows two veins running alongside one artery. This arrangement is commonly found deep within the arms and legs and throughout the entire body. Pressure is applied to the walls of the companion veins by the pulsing of the arteries and contraction of muscles. This pressure forces the blood inside the veins to push through the venous valves and flow toward the heart. The valves prevent blood from flowing backward to the extremities. This is how venous blood in the regions below the level of the heart is sent back to the heart.

6. BLOOD CIRCULATION IN THE FETUS

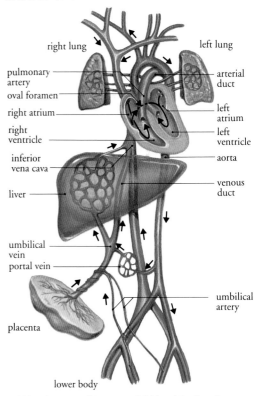

right lung

left lung

pulmonary artery

arterial duct

oval foramen

left atrium

right atrium

right ventricle

left ventricle

inferior vena cava

aorta

liver

venous duct

umbilical vein

portal vein

umbilical artery

placenta

lower body

Fetal blood is turned into arterial blood in the placenta and flows through the venous duct and liver and into the inferior vena cava. In the process, this blood mixes with venous blood from the lower part of the fetal body and enters the right atrium of the heart. This mixed blood flows through a hole in the middle of the atrium called the foramen ovale and into the left atrium. Venous blood from the upper part of the fetal body passes through the right atrium and right ventricle and exits via the pulmonary arteries. Some of this blood is transported to the lungs but most flows through the arterial duct into the aorta.

1. Lymph Nodes of the Head, Neck and Thoracic Regions

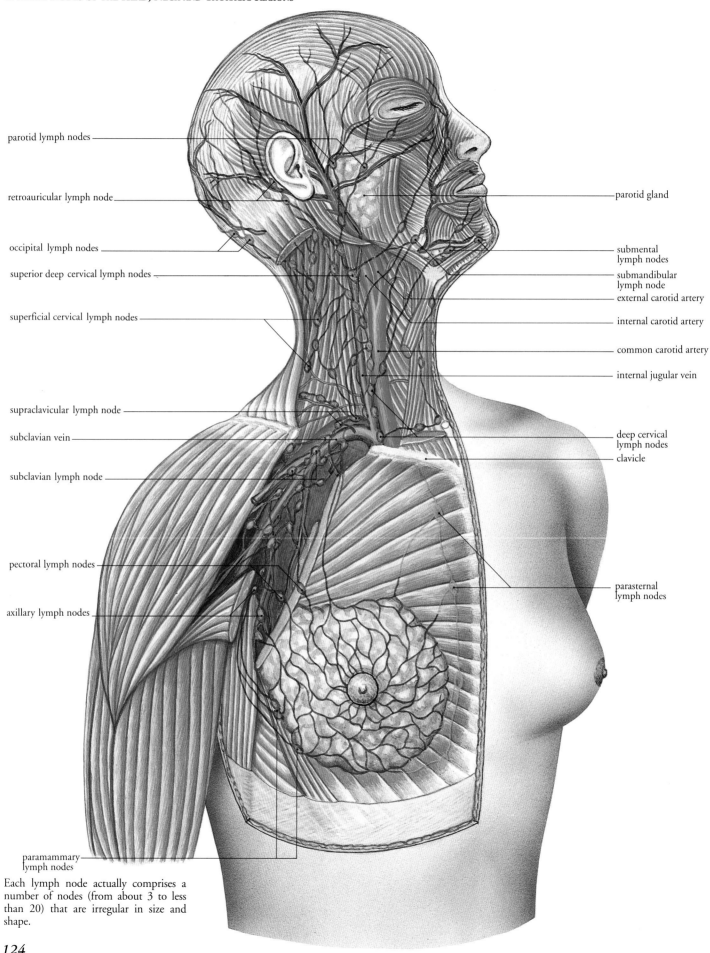

parotid lymph nodes

retroauricular lymph node

occipital lymph nodes

superior deep cervical lymph nodes

superficial cervical lymph nodes

supraclavicular lymph node

subclavian vein

subclavian lymph node

pectoral lymph nodes

axillary lymph nodes

paramammary lymph nodes

parotid gland

submental lymph nodes

submandibular lymph node

external carotid artery

internal carotid artery

common carotid artery

internal jugular vein

deep cervical lymph nodes

clavicle

parasternal lymph nodes

Each lymph node actually comprises a number of nodes (from about 3 to less than 20) that are irregular in size and shape.

2. STRUCTURE OF THE LYMPH NODE

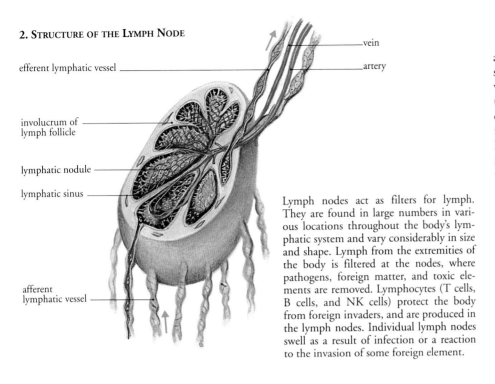

- vein
- artery
- efferent lymphatic vessel
- involucrum of lymph follicle
- lymphatic nodule
- lymphatic sinus
- afferent lymphatic vessel

Lymph nodes act as filters for lymph. They are found in large numbers in various locations throughout the body's lymphatic system and vary considerably in size and shape. Lymph from the extremities of the body is filtered at the nodes, where pathogens, foreign matter, and toxic elements are removed. Lymphocytes (T cells, B cells, and NK cells) protect the body from foreign invaders, and are produced in the lymph nodes. Individual lymph nodes swell as a result of infection or a reaction to the invasion of some foreign element.

3. LYMPH NODES OF THE LOWER LIMBS

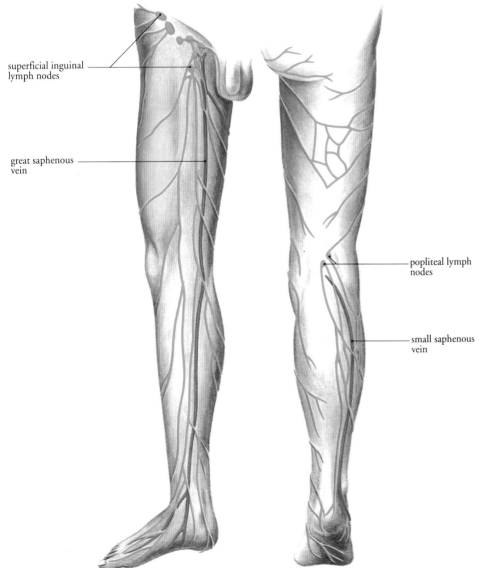

- superficial inguinal lymph nodes
- great saphenous vein
- popliteal lymph nodes
- small saphenous vein

LYMPHATIC VESSELS. Lymphatic vessels and lymph nodes make up the lymphatic system. Resembling a river, the lymphatic vessels begin as microscopic blind ducts (ducts that are closed at the ends) and spread out in a very fine network through body tissue. Lymph, which resembles plasma (the liquid part of blood), enters the vessels by seeping into the lymphatic capillaries. Lymph vessels transport the final by-products of metabolism that have been discharged from the cells, dead cells, blood corpuscles, and bacteria. Lymphocytes, which protect the body against pathogens, are part of the lymph.

Numerous valves are present in the fine ducts close to the ends of lymphatic vessels. These ducts gradually become larger lymph vessels, and along the way numerous nodes filter the lymph. Lymphatic vessels in the head and neck gather at the collection of lymph nodes in the anterior cervical region; those of the arms and chest gather at the lymph nodes under the arms; and those of the lower abdominal area and lower limbs collect at the group of nodes in the inguinal region. The vessels eventually lead into the thoracic duct, which is the main lymphatic pathway, and flow into the veins. The epithelium, cartilage, eyeballs, central nervous system, and spleen have no lymphatic vessels running through them.

LYMPH NODES. The lymph nodes vary in size from microscopic to larger than a bean, and they are oblong or round. Afferent lymphatic vessels bring lymph into the node, and efferent vessels carry lymph out of the node. In the head, arms, and legs, most lymph nodes are close to the surface. In the neck region an equal number of lymph nodes are located near the surface as are deeper within. In the trunk and internal organs, more nodes are located deep beneath the surface. Lymph nodes are not permanent organs but undergo degeneration and regeneration.

Function of the Lymphatic System. The lymphatic system performs the important function of protecting the body from infection by pathogens and other causes. If a wound on the fingertip becomes infected by bacteria, the lymph nodes become swollen and the lymphatic vessels become inflamed and can be seen as red lines in the crook of the arm. If cancer develops, cancer cells flow through the lymphatic vessels and enter the lymph nodes, where they can metastasize. If bacteria overpower the defense capability of lymph, the nodes may be destroyed.

Major Disorders: lymphadenitis, lymphedema.

The Nervous System

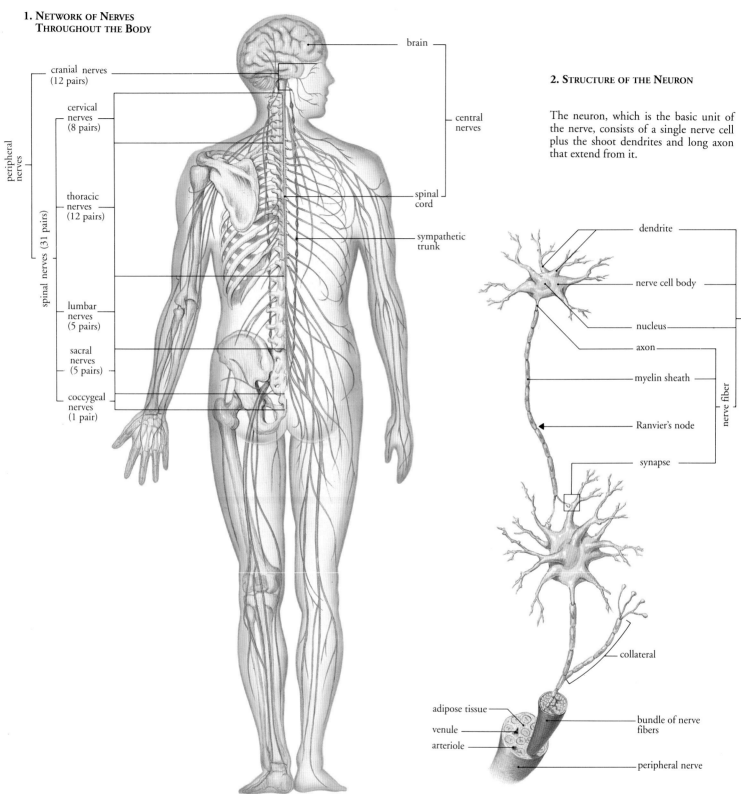

1. NETWORK OF NERVES THROUGHOUT THE BODY

cranial nerves (12 pairs)

cervical nerves (8 pairs)

thoracic nerves (12 pairs)

lumbar nerves (5 pairs)

sacral nerves (5 pairs)

coccygeal nerves (1 pair)

peripheral nerves

spinal nerves (31 pairs)

brain

central nerves

spinal cord

sympathetic trunk

2. STRUCTURE OF THE NEURON

The neuron, which is the basic unit of the nerve, consists of a single nerve cell plus the shoot dendrites and long axon that extend from it.

dendrite

nerve cell body

nucleus

axon

myelin sheath

Ranvier's node

synapse

neuron

nerve fiber

collateral

adipose tissue

venule

arteriole

bundle of nerve fibers

peripheral nerve

The body's nervous system is divided into the central nervous system and the peripheral nervous system. The brain and spinal cord comprise the central nervous system. The brain is the site where mental activity occurs, and the brain and spinal cord together act as the center for maintaining life. The peripheral nervous system is the communication pathway connecting the central nervous system with the various parts of the body (periphery). The peripheral system is divided into the cranial nerves that lead to and from the brain and the spinal nerves that lead to and from the spinal cord. The two systems combined are also known as the cerebrospinal system.

The cranial nerves control feeling and function of the various parts of the head and face, including the muscles, eyes, ears, and nose. The spinal nerves transmit signals from the brain to the four limbs and the trunk and send information from the various parts of the body back to the brain and spinal cord.

The peripheral nervous system is divided into the somatic nervous system (motor and sensory nerves), which receives information from the surface of the body and controls voluntary movement, and the autonomic nervous system, which controls involuntary reactions of the internal organs and blood vessels. The autonomic nervous system works to maintain the internal

A pair of each kind of nerve extends symmetrically left and right from the base of the brain to control a specific region of the body. This figure shows only the cranial nerves of the left side and the areas they control. Roman numerals in parentheses indicate the number of each nerve.

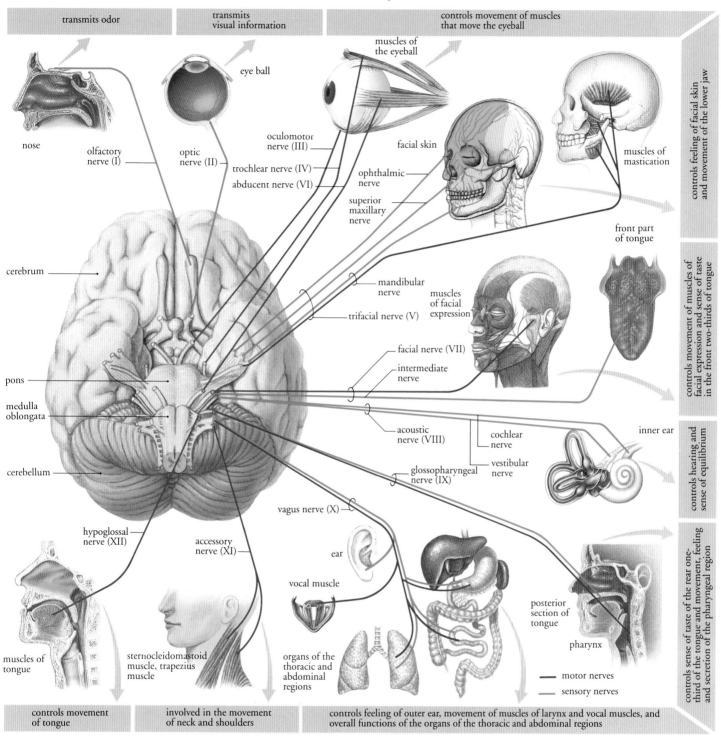

environment of the body through mutual competition between the sympathetic and parasympathetic nervous systems.

CRANIAL NERVES

The cranial nerves are peripheral nerves leading to and from the brain. The 12 pairs of cranial nerves control most functions of the head and face.

The olfactory nerve is responsible for the sense of smell, the optic nerve for the sense of sight, the acoustic nerve for hearing and balance, and the glossopharyngeal nerve and some branches of the facial nerve for the sense of taste. Three pairs of cranial nerves are related to movement of the eyeball and vision: oculomotor, trochlear, and abducent nerves.

The glossopharyngeal nerve controls movement and feeling from the root of the tongue to the pharynx, as well as secretion of saliva. The hypolglossal nerve controls the movement of the tongue. The trifacial nerve controls the general sensory properties of the face as well as the movement of the lower jaw. The vagus nerve controls the movements of the palate, pharynx, and larynx as well as the general functioning of the digestive tract, regulating digestion and uptake of nutrients basic to sustaining life.

The facial nerves control the muscles of facial expression and the accessory nerves move the neck and shoulders, thus playing an important role in giving form to the rich play of emotions unique to human beings.

Major Disorders: facial neuralgia, trifacial neuralgia, facial spasm.

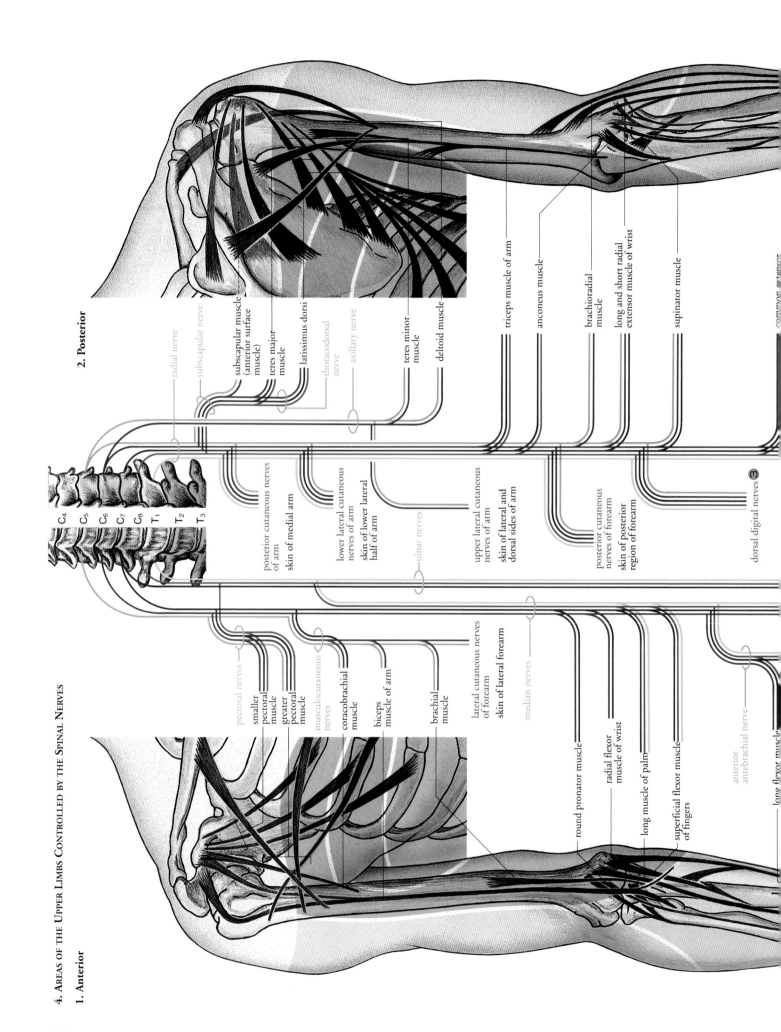

4. AREAS OF THE UPPER LIMBS CONTROLLED BY THE SPINAL NERVES

1. Anterior

2. Posterior

C₄
C₅
C₆
C₇
C₈
T₁
T₂
T₃

radial nerve
subscapular nerve
subscapular muscle (anterior surface muscle)
teres major muscle
latissimus dorsi
thoracodorsal nerve
axillary nerve
teres minor muscle
deltoid muscle

triceps muscle of arm
anconeus muscle
brachioradial muscle
long and short radial extensor muscle of wrist
supinator muscle
common extensor

posterior cutaneous nerves of arm
skin of medial arm
lower lateral cutaneous nerves of arm
skin of lower lateral half of arm
ulnar nerves
upper lateral cutaneous nerves of arm
skin of lateral and dorsal sides of arm
posterior cutaneous nerves of forearm
skin of posterior region of forearm
dorsal digital nerves ③

pectoral nerves
smaller pectoral muscle
greater pectoral muscle
musculocutaneous nerves
coracobrachial muscle
biceps muscle of arm
brachial muscle
lateral cutaneous nerves of forearm
skin of lateral forearm
median nerves
anterior antebrachial nerve

round pronator muscle
radial flexor muscle of wrist
long muscle of palm
superficial flexor muscle of fingers
long flexor muscle

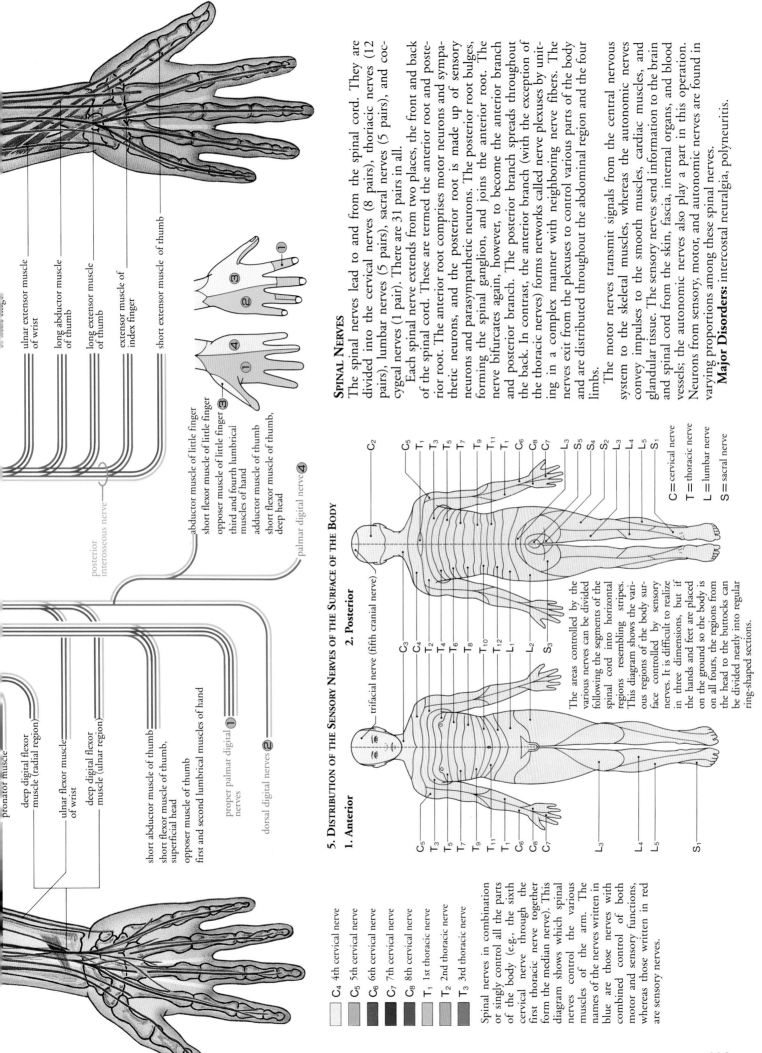

ulnar extensor muscle of wrist

long abductor muscle of thumb

long extensor muscle of thumb

extensor muscle of index finger

short extensor muscle of thumb

posterior interosseous nerve

abductor muscle of little finger
short flexor muscle of little finger
opposer muscle of little finger
third and fourth lumbrical muscles of hand
adductor muscle of thumb
short flexor muscle of thumb, deep head

palmar digital nerve ④

pronator muscle

deep digital flexor muscle (radial region)

ulnar flexor muscle of wrist

deep digital flexor muscle (ulnar region)

short abductor muscle of thumb
short flexor muscle of thumb, superficial head
opposer muscle of thumb
first and second lumbrical muscles of hand

proper palmar digital ① nerves

dorsal digital nerves ②

Spinal nerves in combination or singly control all the parts of the body (eg., the sixth cervical nerve through the first thoracic nerve together form the median nerve). This diagram shows which spinal nerves control the various muscles of the arm. The names of the nerves written in blue are those nerves with combined control of both motor and sensory functions, whereas those written in red are sensory nerves.

C₄ 4th cervical nerve
C₅ 5th cervical nerve
C₆ 6th cervical nerve
C₇ 7th cervical nerve
C₈ 8th cervical nerve
T₁ 1st thoracic nerve
T₂ 2nd thoracic nerve
T₃ 3rd thoracic nerve

5. DISTRIBUTION OF THE SENSORY NERVES OF THE SURFACE OF THE BODY

1. Anterior

2. Posterior

trifacial nerve (fifth cranial nerve)

C₂ C₅ T₁ T₃ T₅ T₇ T₉ T₁₁ T₁ C₆ C₈ C₇ L₃ S₅ S₄ S₂ L₃ L₄ L₅ S₁

C₃ C₄ T₂ T₄ T₆ T₈ T₁₀ T₁₂ L₁ L₂ S₃

C₅ T₃ T₅ T₇ T₉ T₁₁ T₁ C₆ C₈ C₇

L₃ L₄ L₅ S₁

C = cervical nerve
T = thoracic nerve
L = lumbar nerve
S = sacral nerve

The areas controlled by the various nerves can be divided following the segments of the spinal cord into horizontal regions resembling stripes. This diagram shows the various regions of the body surface controlled by sensory nerves. It is difficult to realize in three dimensions, but if the hands and feet are placed on the ground so the body is on all fours, the regions from the head to the buttocks can be divided neatly into regular ring-shaped sections.

SPINAL NERVES

The spinal nerves lead to and from the spinal cord. They are divided into the cervical nerves (8 pairs), thoriacic nerves (12 pairs), lumbar nerves (5 pairs), sacral nerves (5 pairs), and coccygeal nerves (1 pair). There are 31 pairs in all.

Each spinal nerve extends from two places, the front and back of the spinal cord. These are termed the anterior root and posterior root. The anterior root comprises motor neurons and sympathetic neurons, and the posterior root is made up of sensory neurons and parasympathetic neurons. The posterior root bulges, forming the spinal ganglion, and joins the anterior root. The nerve bifurcates again, however, to become the anterior branch and posterior branch. The posterior branch spreads throughout the back. In contrast, the anterior branch (with the exception of the thoracic nerves) forms networks called nerve plexuses by uniting in a complex manner with neighboring nerve fibers. The nerves exit from the plexuses to control various parts of the body and are distributed throughout the abdominal region and the four limbs.

The motor nerves transmit signals from the central nervous system to the skeletal muscles, whereas the autonomic nerves convey impulses to the smooth muscles, cardiac muscles, and glandular tissue. The sensory nerves send information to the brain and spinal cord from the skin, fascia, internal organs, and blood vessels; the autonomic nerves also play a part in this operation. Neurons from sensory, motor, and autonomic nerves are found in varying proportions among these spinal nerves.

Major Disorders: intercostal neuralgia, polyneuritis.

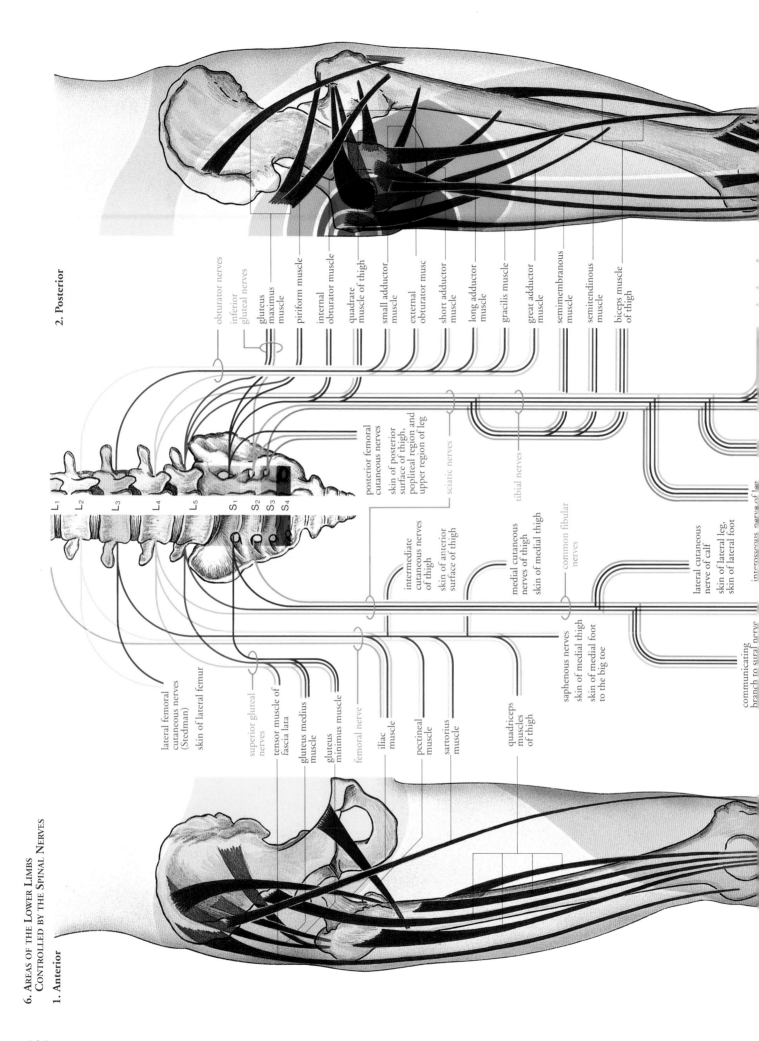

2. Posterior

obturator nerves
inferior gluteal nerves
gluteus maximus muscle
piriform muscle
internal obturator muscle
quadrate muscle of thigh
small adductor muscle
external obturator musc
short adductor muscle
long adductor muscle
gracilis muscle
great adductor muscle
semimembranous muscle
semitendinous muscle
biceps muscle of thigh

posterior femoral cutaneous nerves
skin of posterior surface of thigh, popliteal region and upper region of leg
sciatic nerves
tibial nerves
common fibular nerves
lateral cutaneous nerve of calf
skin of lateral leg, skin of lateral foot
interosseous nerve of leg

intermediate cutaneous nerves of thigh
skin of anterior surface of thigh
medial cutaneous nerves of thigh
skin of medial thigh
saphenous nerves
skin of medial thigh
skin of medial foot to the big toe
communicating branch to sural nerve

lateral femoral cutaneous nerves (Stedman)
skin of lateral femur
superior gluteal nerves
tensor muscle of fascia lata
gluteus medius muscle
gluteus minimus muscle
femoral nerve
iliac muscle
pectineal muscle
sartorius muscle
quadriceps muscles of thigh

L1
L2
L3
L4
L5
S1
S2
S3
S4

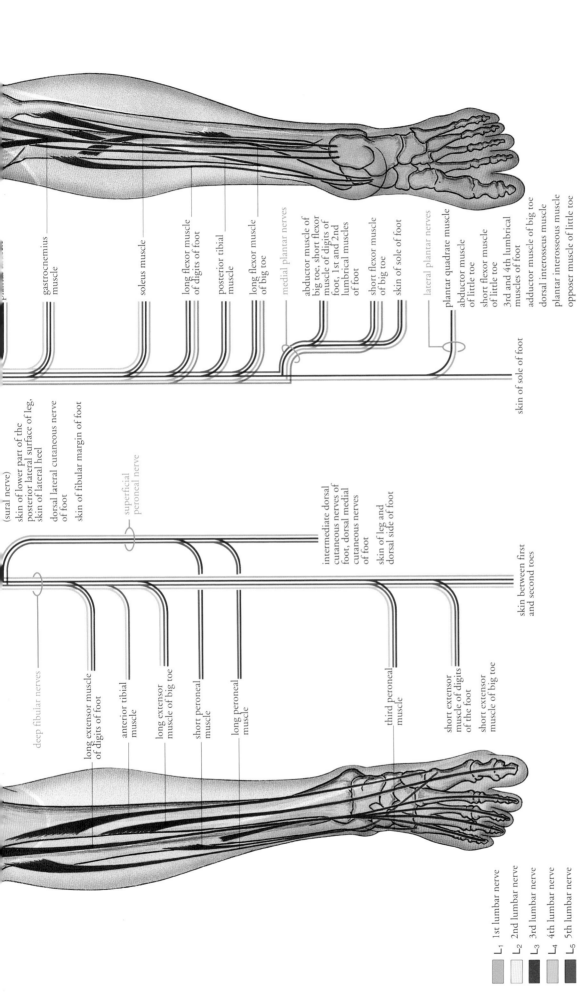

gastrocnemius muscle

soleus muscle

long flexor muscle of digits of foot

posterior tibial muscle

long flexor muscle of big toe

medial plantar nerves

abductor muscle of big toe, short flexor muscle of digits of foot, 1st and 2nd lumbrical muscles of foot

short flexor muscle of big toe

skin of sole of foot

lateral plantar nerves

plantar quadrate muscle

abductor muscle of little toe

short flexor muscle of little toe

3rd and 4th lumbrical muscles of foot

adductor muscle of big toe

dorsal interosseus muscle

plantar interosseous muscle

opposer muscle of little toe

skin of sole of foot

(sural nerve)

skin of lower part of the posterior lateral surface of leg, skin of lateral heel

dorsal lateral cutaneous nerve of foot

skin of fibular margin of foot

superficial peroneal nerve

intermediate dorsal cutaneous nerves of foot, dorsal medial cutaneous nerves of foot

skin of leg and dorsal side of foot

skin between first and second toes

deep fibular nerves

long extensor muscle of digits of foot

anterior tibial muscle

long extensor muscle of big toe

short peroneal muscle

long peroneal muscle

third peroneal muscle

short extensor muscle of digits of the foot

short extensor muscle of big toe

L₁ 1st lumbar nerve

L₂ 2nd lumbar nerve

L₃ 3rd lumbar nerve

L₄ 4th lumbar nerve

L₅ 5th lumbar nerve

S₁ 1st sacral nerve

S₂ 2nd sacral nerve

S₃ 3rd sacral nerve

S₄ 4th sacral nerve

This diagram shows which spinal nerves control the various muscles and skin of the lower limbs. The names of the nerves labeled in blue indicate those nerves combining both motor and sensory functions and the red labels indicate the sensory nerves.

RELATIONSHIP BETWEEN THE AUTONOMIC NERVES AND THE PERIPHERAL NERVES

The autonomic nerves are those that regulate involuntary movement, including movements of the heart, blood vessels, sweat glands, erector muscles of the hair, glandular tissue of the internal organs, and smooth muscles. Although both are part of the peripheral nervous system, the somatic nervous system (motor and sensory nerves) controls the reactions of the body to the external environment, whereas the autonomic nervous system is responsible for regulating the body's internal environment.

The core of the autonomic nervous system is the cell body of the neuron. When an impulse is transmitted to the periphery it must pass a break in the pathway. The neuron that connects the cell body to the ganglion is called the preganglionic fiber and the neuron that joins the ganglion to the peripheral organ is called the postganglionic fiber. In the sympathetic nervous system, the postganglionic fibers are long, because the distance between the sympathetic trunk to which the ganglions are attached and the autonomic plexuses to the organs regulated by the nerves is large. In contrast, in the parasympathetic nervous system the postganglionic fibers are short, because the ganglia are close to the organs.

131

AUTONOMIC NERVOUS SYSTEM

Center of the Autonomic Nervous System. The center of the autonomic nervous system is located in the hypothalamus of the diencephalon, which is covered by the cerebrum. Of the nerve cell layers designated a, b, and c, a and c are the centers of the parasympathetic nervous system, and b is the center for the sympathetic nervous system. The impulses sent out from these centers travel to the preganglionic fiber neurons (page 126) of the midbrain, medulla oblongata, and spinal cord. At the ganglionic connections (synapse) the impulses cross over to a different neuron (postganglionic fiber) and reach the appropriate peripheral organ.

Distribution of the Sympathetic Nervous System. Sympathetic nerve cells are located in the gray and white matter of the spinal cord. Sympathetic trunk ganglia (preganglionic fibers) lead from the spinal cord to the head and organs of the thorax. Those that lead to the internal organs of the abdominal region are the celiac and mesenteric ganglia. These ganglia cross synapses to become postganglionic fibers, which then extend to the various areas they control.

Distribution of the Parasympathetic Nervous System. Nerve cells are located in the midbrain, medulla oblongata, and spinal cord. At the ganglia that are situated close to the organs they control, the preganglionic fibers become postganglionic fibers, and then enter the appropriate organ. The vagus nerve (cranial nerve) passes from the head through the thoracic region and enters the abdominal area where it extends throughout the internal organs of the region. The nerves that lead out from the sacrum are distributed throughout the lower part of the large intestine, bladder, and reproductive organs. Those that extend from the thoracic and lumbar segments spread throughout the blood vessels, muscles, and sweat glands of the body.

Function of the Autonomic Nervous System. Almost all organs are controlled by both the sympathetic and parasympathetic nervous systems. When the appropriate sympathetic nerves transmit the command impulse, heart function is stimulated, blood vessels contract, pupils widen, or gastric function is suppressed. When the appropriate parasympathetic nerve operates, the exact opposite occurs in each case. These mutually opposite functions are the result of balanced commands sent out by the two nervous systems, which manage the internal environment of the body automatically on an involuntary basis. Emotions can have a subtle effect on the working of these two systems, however.

Major Disorders: autonomic imbalance.

1. Sympathetic Nerves

7. Function of the Autonomous Nervous System

The autonomic nervous system is made up of the sympathetic and parasympathetic nervous systems. This diagram shows how the sympathetic and parasympathetic nerves are distributed throughout the various organs.

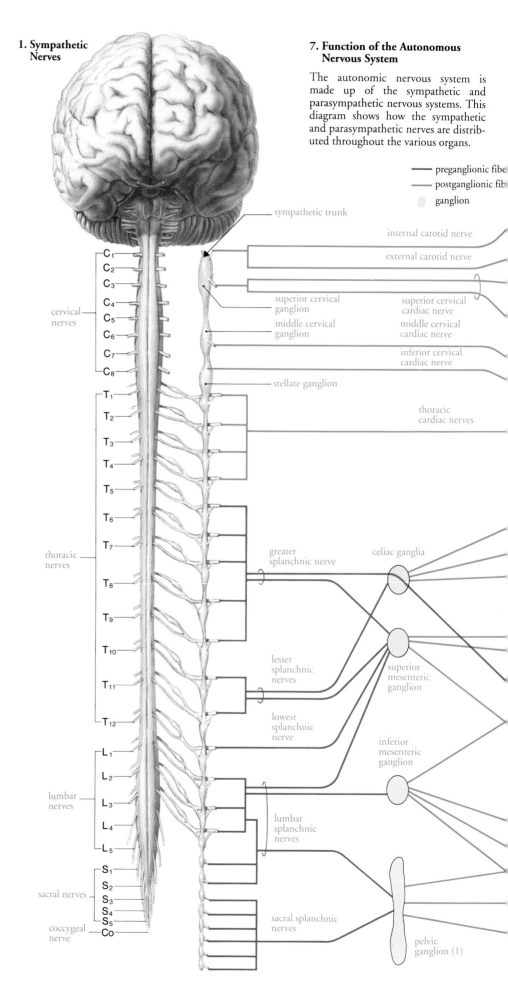

— preganglionic fiber
— postganglionic fiber
▨ ganglion

sympathetic trunk
internal carotid nerve
external carotid nerve
superior cervical ganglion
superior cervical cardiac nerve
middle cervical ganglion
middle cervical cardiac nerve
inferior cervical cardiac nerve
stellate ganglion
thoracic cardiac nerves
greater splanchnic nerve
celiac ganglia
lesser splanchnic nerves
superior mesenteric ganglion
lowest splanchnic nerve
inferior mesenteric ganglion
lumbar splanchnic nerves
sacral splanchnic nerves
pelvic ganglion (1)

cervical nerves
C1 C2 C3 C4 C5 C6 C7 C8
thoracic nerves
T1 T2 T3 T4 T5 T6 T7 T8 T9 T10 T11 T12
lumbar nerves
L1 L2 L3 L4 L5
sacral nerves
S1 S2 S3 S4 S5
coccygeal nerve
Co

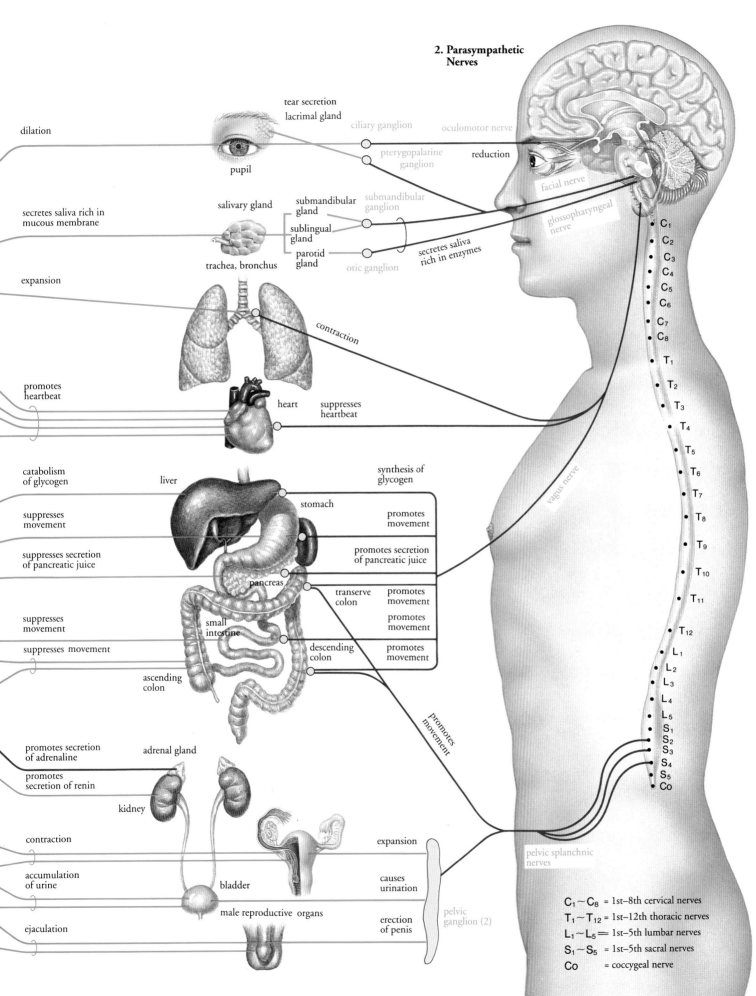

2. Parasympathetic Nerves

dilation

tear secretion
lacrimal gland

ciliary ganglion

oculomotor nerve

pupil

pterygopalatine ganglion

reduction

secretes saliva rich in mucous membrane

salivary gland

submandibular gland

submandibular ganglion

sublingual gland

parotid gland

secretes saliva rich in enzymes

facial nerve

glossopharyngeal nerve

otic ganglion

trachea, bronchus

expansion

contraction

C_1
C_2
C_3
C_4
C_5
C_6
C_7
C_8

T_1
T_2
T_3
T_4
T_5
T_6
T_7
T_8
T_9
T_{10}
T_{11}
T_{12}

promotes heartbeat

heart

suppresses heartbeat

catabolism of glycogen

liver

synthesis of glycogen

stomach

promotes movement

suppresses movement

suppresses secretion of pancreatic juice

promotes secretion of pancreatic juice

pancreas

transerve colon

promotes movement

suppresses movement

small intestine

promotes movement

suppresses movement

descending colon

promotes movement

ascending colon

vagus nerve

L_1
L_2
L_3
L_4
L_5

S_1
S_2
S_3
S_4
S_5
Co

promotes movement

promotes secretion of adrenaline

adrenal gland

promotes secretion of renin

kidney

contraction

expansion

pelvic splanchnic nerves

accumulation of urine

bladder

causes urination

male reproductive organs

ejaculation

erection of penis

pelvic ganglion (2)

$C_1 \sim C_8$ = 1st–8th cervical nerves
$T_1 \sim T_{12}$ = 1st–12th thoracic nerves
$L_1 \sim L_5$ = 1st–5th lumbar nerves
$S_1 \sim S_5$ = 1st–5th sacral nerves
Co = coccygeal nerve

The Endocrine Organs and Hormones

The endocrine glands secrete hormones, substances that transmit humoral information (commands) throughout the body. Communication between the endocrine glands, sexual functions, and functions of the autonomic nervous system are controlled by hormones. The route (circulatory system) of humoral information is naturally separate from the nerve pathway (nervous system), which transmits information via electric impulses, but the two systems influence each other and work to maintain balanced body function.

The pituitary gland of the brain is only about the size of the tip of the small finger, but it plays the role of general manager in regulating the activity of the endocrine system. Among the hormones secreted by the thyroid gland are those that promote metabolism, and the adrenal cortex secretes hormones that relieve physical and mental stress. During puberty, hormones from the gonads prepare the body for adult life, and after puberty, they regulate the processes of reproduction. The placenta produces hormones necessary for the maintenance and growth of the fetus. The islets of Langerhans in the pancreas secrete hormones such as insulin and glucagon, which control sugar metabolism. Parts of the digestive tract, including the stomach and intestines, secrete digestive hormones required for the smooth progress of digestion.

Major Disorders: Addison's disease, diabetes, gigantism, aldosteronism.

DISTRIBUTION OF THE HORMONES OF THE PITUITARY AND OTHER MAJOR ENDOCRINE GLANDS

1. Hypothalamus and Pituitary Gland

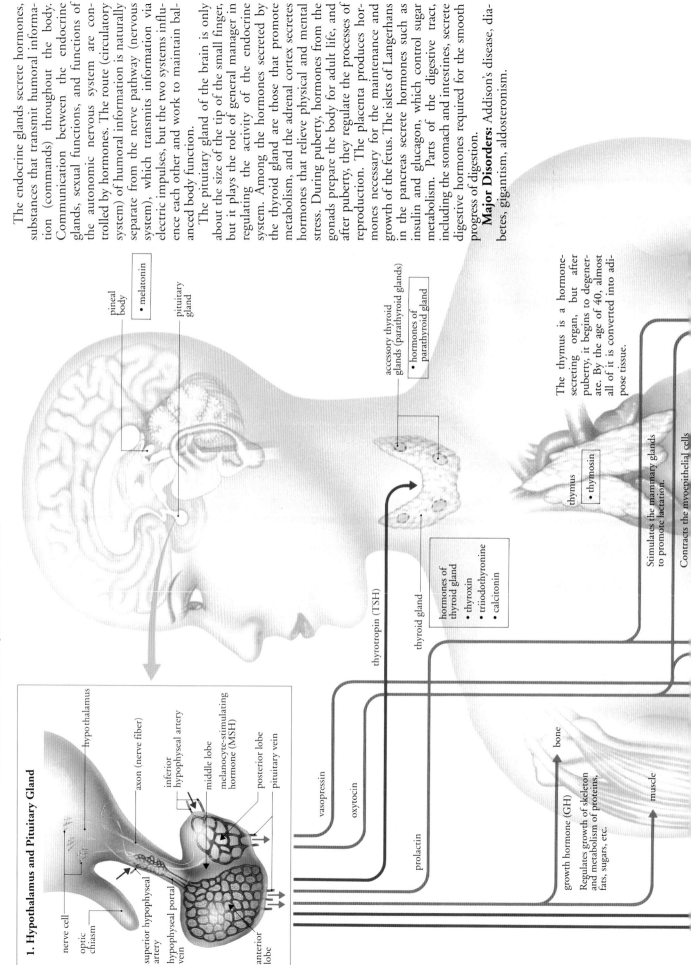

pineal body
• melatonin

pituitary gland

accessory thyroid glands (parathyroid glands)
• hormones of parathyroid gland

hormones of thyroid gland
• thyroxin
• triiodothyronine
• calcitonin

thyrotropin (TSH)

thyroid gland

vasopressin

oxytocin

prolactin

growth hormone (GH)

Regulates growth of skeleton and metabolism of proteins, fats, sugars, etc.

bone

muscle

hypothalamus

axon (nerve fiber)

inferior hypophyseal artery

middle lobe

melanocyte-stimulating hormone (MSH)

posterior lobe

pituitary vein

nerve cell

optic chiasm

superior hypophyseal artery

hypophyseal portal vein

anterior lobe

The thymus is a hormone-secreting organ, but after puberty, it begins to degenerate. By the age of 40, almost all of it is converted into adipose tissue.

thymus
• thymosin

Stimulates the mammary glands to promote lactation.

Contracts the myoepithelial cells

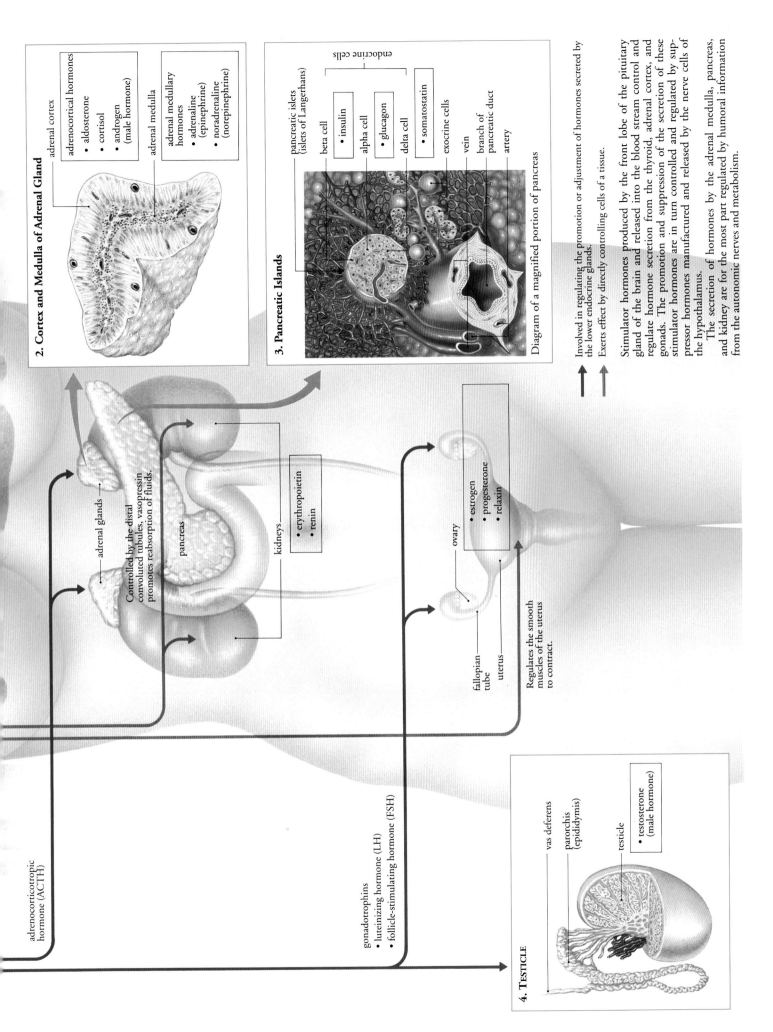

2. Cortex and Medulla of Adrenal Gland

adrenal cortex

adrenocortical hormones
- aldosterone
- cortisol
- androgen (male hormone)

adrenal medulla

adrenal medullary hormones
- adrenaline (epinephrine)
- noradrenaline (norepinephrine)

3. Pancreatic Islands

endocrine cells

pancreatic islets (islets of Langerhans)

beta cell
- insulin

alpha cell
- glucagon

delta cell
- somatostatin

exocrine cells

vein

branch of pancreatic duct

artery

Diagram of a magnified portion of pancreas

↑ Involved in regulating the promotion or adjustment of hormones secreted by the lower endocrine glands.

↑ Exerts effect by directly controlling cells of a tissue.

Stimulator hormones produced by the front lobe of the pituitary gland of the brain and released into the blood stream control and regulate hormone secretion from the thyroid, adrenal cortex, and gonads. The promotion and suppression of the secretion of these stimulator hormones are in turn controlled and regulated by suppressor hormones manufactured and released by the nerve cells of the hypothalamus.

The secretion of hormones by the adrenal medulla, pancreas, and kidney are for the most part regulated by humoral information from the autonomic nerves and metabolism.

adrenocorticotropic hormone (ACTH)

adrenal glands

Controlled by the distal convoluted tubules, vasopressin promotes reabsorption of fluids.

pancreas

kidneys
- erythropoietin
- renin

gonadotrophins
- luteinizing hormone (LH)
- follicle-stimulating hormone (FSH)

ovary
- estrogen
- progesterone
- relaxin

fallopian tube

uterus

Regulates the smooth muscles of the uterus to contract.

4. Testicle

vas deferens

parorchis (epididymis)

testicle
- testosterone (male hormone)

135

Index